Massage and Aromatherapy

A Practical Approach

2nd Edition

Lyn Goldberg

First published in 1995 by:
Stanley Thornes (Publishers) Ltd

Second edition published in 2001 by:
Nelson Thornes Ltd
Delta Place
27 Bath Road
CHELTENHAM
GL53 7TH
United Kingdom

01 02 03 04 05 / 10 9 8 7 6 5 4 3 2 1

A catalogue record for this book is available from the British Library

ISBN 0 7487 5875 5

Line illustrations by Angela Lumley, Oxford Illustrators

Typeset by Florence Production Ltd, Stoodleigh, Devon
Printed and bound in Italy by G. Canale & C.S.p.A, Borgaro T.se, Turin

Contents

ACKNOWLEDGEMENTS

I am indebted to the following for their help and advice during the preparation of this edition:

Carlton Professional and New Concept for their generousity in supplying photographs of couches and equipment; Marion Campbell of The London College of Fashion for her advice on aromatherapy and Eastern techniques; Claire Hart at Nelson Thornes for help and support when I needed it; and my husband and daughters for their tolerance and expertise.

INTRODUCTION

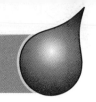

In recent years there has been an amazing increase in the use of massage as a therapy. Until fairly recently any mention of massage other than that used in osteopathy or physiotherapy to treat some medical conditions was regarded with deep suspicion. The growth and acceptance of therapies complementary to orthodox medicine have led to massage being much more widely accepted as a treatment for all sorts of stress-related problems. Of course massage in one form or another has been used in this country and in most parts of the world since time immemorial, but only now in Britain is it becoming so widely accepted that many men and women are training and becoming professional massage therapists outside the medical field.

The English word 'massage' is probably derived from the Arabic *mass'h* meaning to press softly.

There can hardly be a culture where rubbing or pressing of some sort has not been part of the healing process in the past and in many of them the tradition continues alongside the practice of modern medicine. Very often aromatic oils and herbal remedies have been used with massage to help the healing process and we see a revival of this today in the practice of aromatherapy.

We must assume that just as man found food by trial and error and by an instinctive recognition of his needs, so in illness he must have found some substances which acted as drugs to help fend off disease. Many ancient peoples possessed a considerable knowledge of such substances, which was passed down from father to son, or more likely from mother to daughter as it was they who prepared food and therefore knew how to prepare a healing potion. Instinct must also have played a large part in the development of physical treatments as instinctive rubbing of a sore part of the body is found to relieve pain or discomfort, this rubbing, developed into a system, becomes massage.

Records show that massage was practised in China as early as 3000 BC with one of the earliest books containing a list of exercises and massage movements. Their techniques concentrated on finding points on the body where pressing and rubbing were most effective. These techniques spread to Japan and have developed into the system known today as shiatsu.

In many American Indian tribes, traditional medicine was based on the idea that disease was the result of objects which had become embedded in the body and that removing them would help the problem. The medicine men had many methods of appearing to remove them and often preceded these magical routines by rubbing movements which themselves were pain relieving. The Navahos held lengthy healing ceremonials which would combine all the elements of 'primitive' medicine, religious prayers and dances, magic items such as sand paintings and sticks but also more rational treatments such as sweat baths, incense, drugs and massage.

Massage is referred to in ancient Hindu books such as the *Ayurveda* (Art of Life) which dates from 1800 BC. In Indian villages today there is usually someone expert in massage who will often combine massage treatments with the use of herbs, spices and aromatic oils.

Various forms of massage were used in the middle east and there are letters from as early as the 7th century BC from a physician in Assyria giving instructions for treatment of his king by applying herbs and vigorous massage until he perspired.

Other cultures with documented references to massage are found in Indonesia, Australia and Tahiti. Captain Cook is said to have been cured of sciatica when Tahitan women used massage on him.

In Europe there is a long history of the use of massage, in Ancient Greece and Rome it was used to revive soldiers and gladiators and was part of the regular lifestyle of wealthy citizens. Physical fitness was very important to the Ancient Greeks with regular competitive races and gymnastic displays being held. Regular massage was prescribed for the athletes to keep them supple and fit. Homer, in the *Odyssey*, refers to massage with nutrition and exercise to promote healing and fitness for soldiers. Greek women are known to have used gymnastics, dancing and massage as part of their beauty regime. The Greek physician Herodicus, in the 5th century BC, used herbs and oils with massage and his pupil Hippocrates recognised the efficacy of stroking movements towards the heart long before the circulation of the blood was understood. Hippocrates advised physicians to learn massage as 'rubbing can bind and loosen, can make flesh and cause parts to waste; hard rubbing binds, soft rubbing loosens; much rubbing causes parts to waste, moderate rubbing makes them grow.'

The Romans probably acquired the practice of massage and baths from the Greeks and practitioners followed the directions of Hippocrates. The Roman system of baths played a large part in the life of wealthy citizens. The baths were taken in four stages, first a gradual warming up, then a much hotter bath leading to profuse sweating, which was followed by cooling down in a tepid bath and then a cold plunge. During each stage slaves rubbed down the bathers often using brushes and bone utensils to scrape the skin.

Galen, a noted Roman physician of the 1st century AD who discovered that the arteries contained blood, recommended massage for treatment of injury and disease with the strokes being varied in direction according to the result required. The techniques mentioned in Roman times include pummelling, pinching and squeezing. Julius Caesar is said to have had himself rubbed and pinched all over each day to help his neuralgia.

There are occasional references to massage as a beauty treatment in the Middle Ages but not much was heard of it from the medical world until the 1570s when Ambroise Pare, a French surgeon, reported that he used friction movements to reduce swelling before treating dislocations of joints. He is known to have classified movements into gentle, medium and vigorous and is credited with successfully treating Mary Queen of Scots with massage.

Over the next three centuries more was heard of massage and in 1700, in Prussia, the King's physician Hoffman used it with exercise to treat his aristocratic patients. By 1800, an Oxford surgeon, John Grosvenor, was using friction to ease stiff joints and a Mr Balfour of Edinburgh used rubbing, percussion and compression for rheumatism and gout. It was a Swedish physiologist Peter Henry Ling who developed a clear system of massage and exercise in the early 1800s and whose terminology is still used today to describe Swedish-style massage. The terms 'effleurage', 'petrissage' and 'vibration' were used by him as well as 'friction', 'rolling' and 'slapping'. By the middle of the 19th century French, German and Dutch physicians were modernising and changing the old skills of rubbing and adopting Ling's methods.

It was a Dutch physician, Dr Johann Metzger, who established massage as part of medical practice. In 1860 he cured the Danish crown prince of a joint infection and developed his methods to agree with the current knowledge of anatomy and physiology. Holland was the first European country to have a massage organisation and journal and many other Dutch physicians carried on Metzger's work. He had followers in other countries including America but it was his German followers, especially a Professor von Mosengeil, who promoted his theories in Britain. In the *British Medical Journal* of May 1866, Dr William Murrell published an article on 'Massage as a Therapeutic Agent' referring to its use by German doctors and by a Dr Graham of the Massachusetts Therapeutic Massage Association. Dr Graham claimed to have developed methods of treatments which were later used by a German calligrapher called Julius Wolff. This was a way of treating writer's cramp with massage and exercise which was so successful that his method was widely accepted by British doctors. He is also known to have influenced such famous French physicians as Charcot and Lucas-Champonnière. In 1889, Lucas-Champonnière published his book *Massage and Mobilisation in the Treatment of Fractures.*

By the late 1800s, British doctors were advocating that nurses should be trained in massage to be used in the medical field and in 1894 a group of women founded the Society of Trained Masseuses. These women while having nursing backgrounds were interested in developing and regulating physical treatments which, as we have seen, has roots going back into ancient history.

In about 1885, there was an article published in a manual called *The Family Physician* which was a warning from doctors to the general public about massage as a career for young women. This said that there was no demand for people to train as masseuses and that the only people likely to make an income from it are 'the not over scrupulous people who give lessons and persuade unwary women that it is lucrative employment'. The article also pointed out that at that time there was no body or corporation with authority to issue qualifications in massage so that the certificates issued by teachers were valueless. Warning was given too about the unsavoury nature of some so-called massage establishments which were advertised in the fashionable London papers.

The Society of Trained Masseuses flourished with membership increasing during the First World War. A Royal Charter was granted in 1920 and it became the Chartered Society of Massage and Medical

Gymnastics. The name was changed again in 1943 to the Chartered Society of Physiotherapy with state registration in 1964. So it was that the use of massage was effectively kept as part of the medical establishment for many years until physiotherapists asserted their professional independence by which time massage was used much less in hospitals.

Following the decline of massage as a treatment for medical conditions there was an increase in its use as part of 'holistic' treatments outside the orthodox medical establishment. Holism is defined in the 1990 *Oxford English Dictionary* as 'The treating of the whole person including mental and social factors rather than just symptoms of disease'. Many practitioners are now involved in this alternative view of health care working in clinics, health centres, fitness centres and others using many different titles.

This recent popularity of complementary therapies has created an interest in massage once again by nurses and other health care professionals. There is a desire by many to return to a more caring role alongside the medical model that has dominated their work in past years.

The skill of massage allows nurses to touch patients therapeutically in a way that allows meaningful communication between them. The importance of touch in caring for people, particularly the elderly and confused, has been shown to promote trust and empathy apart from any physical benefits gained from treatments. However, it is most important to realise that clients or patients may not want to be touched in this way and may feel threatened by an inapproprite approach. This can usually be overcome by careful explanation of the process. Massage is also being used to help patients with conditions believed to be caused by stress and which are made worse by anxiety.

Aromatherapy using massage and aromatic essential oils is also gaining acceptance in some hospitals and clinics where relaxation is seen as a priority. Nurses in training now may be offered some training in massage and in Germany aromatherapy is part of the curriculum for every student nurse.

Massage plays a significant part in beauty therapy training and apart from full body massage, is incorporated into many treatments. In facial work, massage movements will be used in cleansing and most other face and skin treatments. In a pedicure treatment, massage movements will be used to apply lotions and to stimulate the circulation and relax the feet and lower legs. Massage has gradually become a larger part of the beauty therapist's work with the increase in the public's interest in complementary therapies. In 1968, the first full-time nationally recognised course in beauty therapy was offered in a college of further education by the City and Guilds of London Institute and many other organisations now offer full training courses.

Massage and aromatherapy massage is now included in many courses under the auspices of the National Council for Vocational Qualifications (NCVQ) and other organisations. These courses allow massage therapists, beauty therapists, nurses and others to acquire nationally recognised, free-standing qualifications in both of these skills. There are also many courses run by private organisations which give excellent qualifications within the context of complementary therapies.

Massage and aromatherapy may be studied as a full- or part-time course at any level, from an evening class to a three-year degree, towards a career or as an extra interest. This book should be suitable for students following any massage and aromatherapy courses, particularly the following:

- Edexcel (BTEC) National Diploma in Applied Science (Beauty Therapy)
- Edexcel (BTEC) Level 3 Complementary Medicine Award
- Edexcel (BTEC) Higher National Diploma in Beauty Therapy and Health Studies
- NVQ/SVQ in Beauty Therapy, Units 305 & 307.

Nurses and health care workers with an interest in complementary therapies will also find this book useful.

Massage and Aromatherapy courses are run by many awarding bodies, including the following:

- International Therapy Examination Council (ITEC)
- Guild of Complementary Practitioners (GCP)
- Vocational Training Charitable Trust (VTCT)
- International Federation of Aromatherapists (IFA)
- International Society of Professional Aromatherapists (ISPA).

Finally, a note on Key Skills: the Key Skills qualificiation will be something that most, if not all of you, will have experience of if you are in training for the workplace. Key skills are the elements of your study that relate to Communication, Application of Number and Information Technology. There may be numerous instances where you make use of these skills but the following are a few examples.

- *Communication* may be centered around consultation: receiving and recording information from clients, on-going communication with clients, developing consultation documents and group discussion of the value of different aspects of consultation.
- *Application of Number* may be centred around business skills: comparative costing of rentals, of equipment and of materials, pricing of treatments, keeping balance sheets, working out profits and controlling stock.
- *Information Technology* may be assessed in many areas: word processing skills in developing consultation documents, client records and advertising leaflets (importing graphics); development of databases of suppliers of equipment and products; and Internet searches of professional organisations and suppliers.

Lyn Goldberg
MCSP, Grad. Dip. Phys., MRQA

THE MASSAGE THERAPIST IN THE WORKPLACE

After working through this chapter you will be able to:
- describe a variety of employment opportunities for massage therapists
- recognise the importance of observing current legislation
- recognise the importance of personal hygiene.

Body massage is used by massage therapists, beauty therapists and complementary therapists for a number of purposes. It can be for relaxation or it may be used in conjunction with creams or lotions that have specific effects on the skin and underlying tissues. Sports therapists use massage to help athletes and sports people to prepare for events and to recover afterwards. Aromatherapists use it as a method of applying essential oils of plants which have their own specific therapeutic effects. General and localised massage is once again being used in hospitals and hospices as part of treatment for the very ill and the very old, not necessarily for specific medical conditions but as part of the caring process. Many nurses and professional carers are training in massage techniques. A great deal of research is taking place designed to see whether recovery rates and the general quality of life can be improved by massage and other complementary therapies.

Types of workplace

The types of centre where massage may be carried out and massage therapists employed have increased with the popularity of massage itself. Beauty salons where facial and body treatments are carried out may include body massage in their slimming or relaxation programmes. Massage, of course, will not make a client lose weight but does help in making the client more body conscious and may act as an incentive to take more care with diet and exercise.

Salons offering the whole range of treatments are now not only found as small businesses but may be part of much larger enterprises. Large department stores will have salons often with associated treatment spas and facilities for complementary therapies. Hotels, especially those in large towns and holiday resorts also have salons which offer treatments to an international clientele. Health farms which in the past were mainly aimed at clients needing to lose weight are now attracting clients in need of relaxation and stress management; massage is the one therapy that is included in almost every client's regime. Many clients who receive massage for the first time at a health farm become regular clients at beauty salons or other centres. Fitness and sports centres will often have a massage or sports therapist on the premises to work with clients before or after their exercise programme.

Many beauty and massage therapists work on a freelance basis visiting clients in their homes or in hospitals and hospices. Some hospitals now employ massage therapists or specially trained nurses to work with patients principally in cardiac and psychiatric wards. In some offices, where there is an effort to reduce stress at work, the staff may receive a shoulder and neck massage at their desks. Even airlines are now recognising that to offer massage and relaxation treatments in their VIP lounges will attract custom.

Good massage or beauty therapists may well find themselves demonstrating and teaching the lay person to massage as classes are now held in many evening institutes alongside exercise and yoga classes. In a salon or fitness centre, clients may be interested to learn massage techniques to use on their babies and children.

There are many opportunities for a good massage therapist. However, with many more people in training and interest in massage increasing, it is becoming very competitive. Success as a massage therapist requires dedication and a lot of hard work.

Wherever massage is carried out, the surroundings must be suitable, hygienic and should ensure privacy as far as is possible. Assuming that massage is to be carried out in a small business or clinic setting all of the following employment standards and legislation apply.

Employment standards and legislation

Health and Safety at Work Act 1974

This Act specifies that the *employer* must:

- safeguard as far as possible the health, safety and welfare of themselves, their employees, contractors' employees and members of the public
- keep all equipment up to standard
- ensure the environment is free from toxic fumes
- have safety equipment checked regularly
- make sure all staff know the safety procedures and provide safety information and training
- ensure safe systems of work.

The *employees* must:

- take reasonable care to avoid injury to themselves and others
- co-operate with others
- not interfere with or misuse anything provided to protect their health and safety.

Fire Precautions Act 1971

- All premises must have fire-fighting equipment in good working order.
- The equipment must be readily available and suitable for the types of fire that are likely to occur.
- Doors should be left unlocked to allow a quick exit in the event of fire.
- Room contents should not obstruct the exits.

The employee should:

- keep flammable materials away from heat
- avoid overloading electrical circuits
- avoid trailing leads
- switch off all electrical appliances after use
- not smoke on the premises.

Electricity at Work Regulations 1990

Every electrical appliance or piece of equipment must be tested at least once a year by a qualified electrician. A written record must be kept of these tests and be available for inspection by the Health and Safety authority.

COSHH: The Control of Substances Hazardous to Health Act 1989

This act requires employers to identify hazardous substances in the workplace and control people's exposure to them. (Most substances used in a salon or clinic are safe under normal circumstances but some, such as cologne and essential oils, are flammable if exposed to naked flames.)

The Employers Liability (Compulsory Insurance) Act 1969

The act requires that employers have everyone on their payroll covered by this insurance and that a current certificate of insurance is displayed at the place of work. The insurance provides cover for claims that might arise when an employee suffers illness or injury as a result of negligence by either the employer or another employee. Employees who are injured as a result of their own negligence are not covered by the act.

Public-liability insurance

Public-liability insurance is not statutory, but is taken out by employers to cover them for claims made by members of the public as a result of injury or damage to personal property caused by the employer or employee at work. A special professional indemnity insurance extends this liability to cover named employees against claims, by clients, of personal injury resulting directly from a treatment. Individual therapists should have insurance through their professional organisation to cover them in case of claims by clients.

ACTIVITY

Check your workplace or college for safety hazards and note the position and type of any fire-fighting equipment.

When a salon, clinic or business is being set up where massage is to be offered commercially, application should be made to the Environmental Services department of the local authority where the establishment is situated. All local authorities issue licences which govern premises and therapists offering certain treatments and some authorities include massage in their list of treatments. Authorities including massage are, in the main, the major metropolitan authorities which have their own bye-laws which must be observed. These prescribe standard conditions for special treatment licences, for example the Birmingham City Council Act 1990 and the London Local Authorities Act 1991. The licences issued are usually for a year, are charged for and allow for inspection by the Environmental Services officers who have the authority to fine or cancel the registration of businesses which do not maintain appropriate standards.

Whether a licence is needed or not you must observe basic rules. You must:

- avoid working on clients if you have a contagious disease or infectious illness
- keep your working area clean and tidy
- maintain high standards of hygiene in all aspects of work
- check that the client is suitable for treatment with no contraindications
- explain the treatment clearly to the client
- take all necessary safety precautions before, during and after treatment
- use correct techniques and never skimp on treatment
- adapt treatment appropriately to suit individual clients
- take care when handling or disposing of substances used
- remove waste and dispose of it as soon as possible
- keep accurate records of treatments given noting any abnormal reactions or problems.

ACTIVITY
Write to the Environmental Services department of your local authority to find out what conditions must be fulfilled in order to carry out massage treatments in your locality.

GOOD PRACTICE

Massage treatment involves close contact with clients and great care must be taken with personal appearance and hygiene.

- Clothing should be clean and comfortable allowing adequate room to move while working.
- Jewellery should be kept to an absolute minimum, especially on the hands.
- Hair should be clean, tidy and off the face.
- Shoes should have low heels and be comfortable.
- Body and breath odour must be avoided.
- Nails should be short and unvarnished.

Key Terms
You need to know what these words mean. Go back through the chapter or check in the glossary to find out.

- Hazards
- Hygienic
- Insurance
- Relaxation
- Therapist

THE WORKING ENVIRONMENT

After working through this chapter you will be able to:

♦ describe the preferred features of the working area
♦ recognise the effect the working environment has on the client and the therapist
♦ describe a variety of beds, couches and supports suitable for use in massage
♦ recognise the importance of suitable equipment
♦ select appropriate beds, couches or supports for the working environment
♦ select suitable bed coverings and other linen and accessories
♦ select massage mediums to suit a variety of clients and massage types.

The working area

As we have seen, a massage therapist may be required to work in many differing environments. However, while massage may be carried out with little or no equipment, a therapist will usually be working in a treatment room specifically set aside for the purpose of massage and related treatments.

Size

A treatment room or cubicle should be large enough to hold the couch and a trolley and to allow the therapist to move freely around the couch.

Decor

A treatment room should be relaxing and welcoming. The working area should preferably have a good supply of natural light. When artificial lighting is needed it should not be too bright and should be indirect so that it does not shine into the client's eyes.

The floor should be of a material that is easily cleaned and maintained but which is not noisy, slippery or too cold.

Temperature and ventilation

The room must be warm enough for the client not to become chilled but not so warm as to make it uncomfortable for the therapist. It should be ventilated to prevent it becoming stuffy.

In warm climates, a quiet method of air-conditioning is ideal but must not be uncomfortably cooling.

Privacy

The cubicle should be fully enclosed with a material that gives complete privacy to the client. If the cubicle has complete walls rather than curtains, then the door to the cubicle should be able to be completely shut, but should not be lockable from inside or outside.

> **REMEMBER**
> Clients can become chilled very easily during massage while the working therapist may feel very warm.

Hygiene

Toilet facilities for clients and staff must be readily available. Within the treatment cubicle, there should be a washbasin with a supply of soap and disposable towels. There may be showering facilities on the premises depending on the other treatments being offered but these are not essential.

Equipment

Trolley

The trolley holds items that will be used during the massage. It should be moveable and have quiet, smooth running castors. It must be easy to clean. It can be quite small as it is required to hold only the items needed during the treatment.

Table or cupboard

A table or cupboard is required for spare pillows, extra linen and any large items that will not fit onto the trolley

Massage couch

There is a tremendous variety of suitable couches available for massage therapy varying from portable, folding couches suitable for small salons or home visits to the latest 'state of the art' adjustable couches. Whichever couch is used, it must be long and wide enough for clients of varying sizes and be absolutely secure. There can be nothing worse than lying on a couch that wobbles and squeaks when receiving a massage that should be relaxing!

GOOD PRACTICE

The height of the couch is important to the therapist: too low and you will have to stoop to work and are quite likely to develop back problems; too high and you have to stretch and will be unable to use your body weight to apply necessary leverage. You should be able to stand by the couch and place the flat of your hand on the couch with a straight arm.

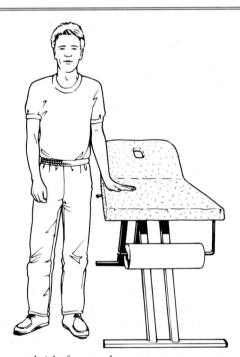

Figure 2.1 *The correct height for a couch*

Adjustable couches, although expensive, are the best for a number of reasons: therapists of differing heights can use them, they can be lowered for elderly or disabled clients who might have difficulty in getting onto a normal height couch and they can be used for differing techniques requiring a lower height such as some sports massage manipulations where greater leverage is required.

Couches of all types will have an adjustable backrest and may have other useful features such as a paper-roll holder and a breathing hole. The breathing hole allows clients to lie face down avoiding the need to turn the head and allows easy access to the back of the neck and shoulders. Couches should be covered in an easily cleaned material such as vinyl and be lightly padded for comfort.

Folding/portable couch

Portable couches can be made to order in a variety of heights to suit a particular therapist. They must be stable with legs that can be locked firmly into the open position. They are often supplied with a carrying case to protect the covering during transit. Such couches are portable in the sense that they can be folded but as they weigh 15 to 17 kg they can be difficult to carry a long way. They are particularly useful for visiting clients in their own homes, for taking to demonstrations or for erecting in a cubicle which is only infrequently used for massage. Some portable couches have legs which can be adjusted to varying heights.

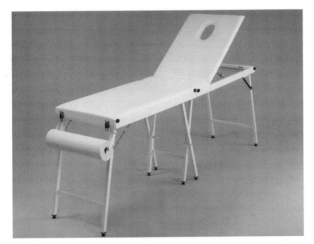

Figure 2.2 *Portable couch: erected*

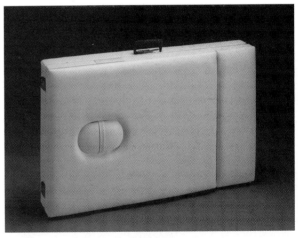

Figure 2.3 *Portable couch: folded*

General purpose massage couch

These couches may have a metal or wooden frame and are the basic couches for massage. They may be suitable for treatments other than massage. Some couches are designed to pack flat and can be reassembled quite quickly if needed.

Multipurpose couch

A multipurpose couch will be suitable for treatments other than massage and will be more versatile than the standard couch. There may be an adjustable foot piece as well as a back support and the central section may allow the shape of the couch to be altered for maximum relaxation and to allow the legs to be raised if necessary.

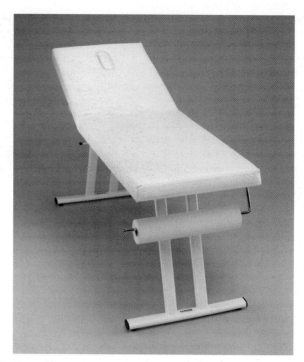

Figure 2.4 *General purpose massage couch*

Hydraulic or electric height-adjustable couch

The couch is raised and lowered by a foot-operated hydraulic pump – similar couches can be operated electrically.

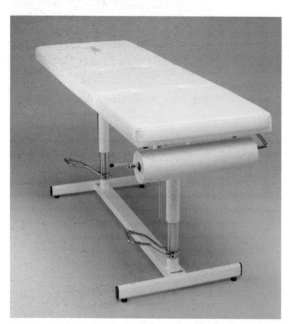

Figure 2.5 *Hydraulic height-adjustable couch: flat*

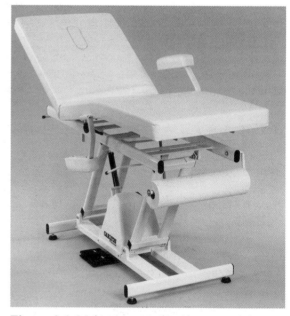

Figure 2.6 *Multipurpose couch with arms and electric lift*

Couch for sports massage

Sports massage requires an extremely firm surface to be effective and ideally the height of the couch should be adjustable. The most important features of all beds and couches for massage are strength and stability.

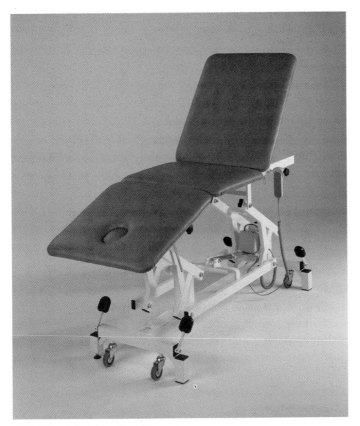

Figure 2.7 *Electric height-adjustable couch*

Support for back massage

For a back massage in the sitting position it may be useful to have a special support which can be propped up on a table to support the client's head and shoulders which is complete in itself. This type of support is often used when visiting clients in the office or other workplace. For a back massage in a kneeling position the special massage chair (shown in Figures 2.9 and 2.10) can be used.

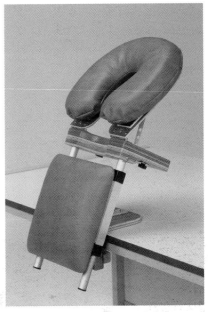

Figure 2.8 *Head and shoulder support*

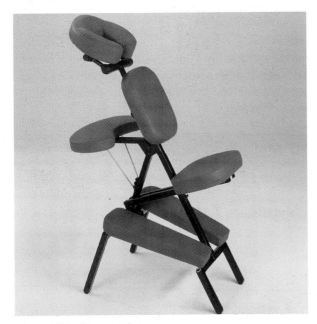

Figure 2.9 *Massage chair*

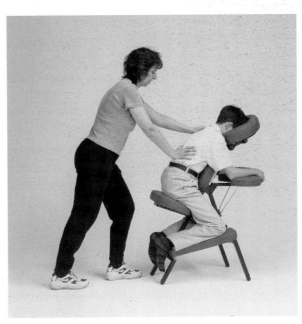

Figure 2.10 *Back massage*

ACTIVITY

By consulting suppliers and catalogues, find out the current cost of each type of couch listed.

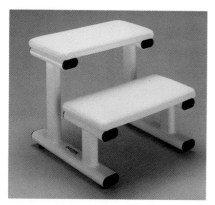

Figure 2.11 *Couch steps*

Steps

A set of steps is useful to allow clients to get on and off the couch more easily. They must be strong and secure and should be stowed away when not in use.

Stool

It is very often convenient to have a stool in the room for the client's or therapist's occasional use during a foot or facial massage.

Accessories

Face cushion

If the couch does not have a breathing hole it will help some clients to use a face cushion which may be inflatable. This allows the client to lie face down in comfort while the therapist is able to work on the back of the neck and shoulders more easily.

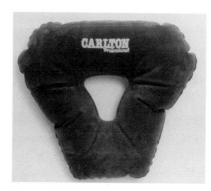

Figure 2.12 *Face cushion*

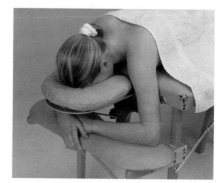

Figure 2.13 *Head rest*

Head, foot and arm rests

There are some extensions available for couches which may be of benefit to use with larger or tall clients. These extensions take the form of a head rest which can be attached to one end of the couch, a foot rest for the other end and arm rests for the sides.

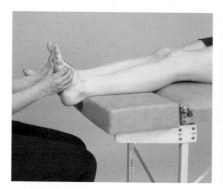

Figure 2.14 *Foot rest*

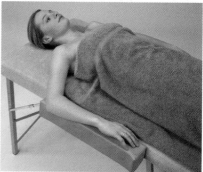

Figure 2.15 *Arm rest*

Linen

There should be a plentiful supply of fresh clean linen and this should include:

- covers for the couch made from elasticised towelling or similar material to fit the couch closely
- pillows (small and full size) and pillow covers
- towels of a variety of sizes
- a light blanket.

The couch may be made up in any convenient way. Commonly, it will have the towelling cover in place and two pillows at head level. These will be covered with disposable paper tissue which is usually kept on a roll at the base of the couch.

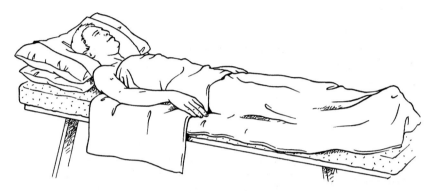

Figure 2.16 *Covering the client*

Two bath-size towels can be used to cover the client, one across the upper half of the body and the other lengthways covering the lower half of the body. This arrangement allows easy access to all parts of the body without too much disturbance.

As the body cools very quickly during massage, a blanket should be on hand to cover the client if necessary.

Small pillows or rolled up towels are useful to support parts of the body during the massage e.g. under the ankle when working on the back of the leg.

Another method of making up the couch is to have a light, flat sheet or blanket on the couch with a covering of disposable paper tissue. The sheet is folded across the client and folded back to expose each area in turn.

Items needed for massage

Items needed for massage should be kept on the moveable trolley so that they are always to hand. These should include:

- massage creams and oils in easily cleaned refillable containers which do not spill
- talcum powder

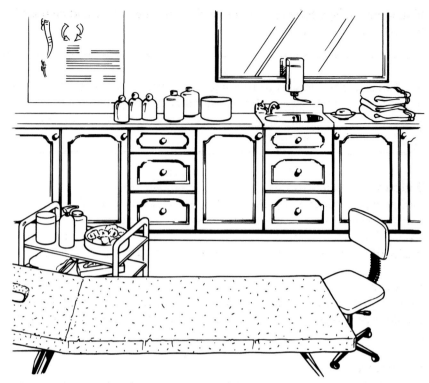

Figure 2.17 *The treatment area*

- cologne
- surgical spirit
- facial cleansers
- tissues
- cotton wool balls or small pads
- bowl or small waste bin for used tissue and cotton wool.

Massage creams and oils

There is a vast range of oils and creams suitable for body massage ranging from mineral oils which are cheap and can be bought in bulk, to proprietary brand named creams and oils which can be very expensive.

Mineral oils

Mineral oils such as baby oils have the disadvantage of not being absorbed easily by the skin and tending to block the pores. They have the advantage of not going rancid – which vegetable oils may do – if kept too long. Mineral oils are particularly suitable for use while learning to massage as they are relatively cheap.

Vegetable oils

Any good-quality vegetable oil may be used such as sunflower, safflower, grapeseed or almond oil. Many therapists use a mixture such as almond oil with a little coconut oil. Care must be taken to keep any vegetable oil fresh and it is a mistake to buy too large an amount at one time. It is best to choose an oil which has little or no smell and is not too thick.

Some commercially produced massage oils or creams may be advised for specific purposes such as treating clients with arthritic complaints or localised cellulite or stretch marks.

If an aromatherapy massage is to be carried out, the oils should be mixed for each individual client.

Talcum powder

Occasionally a client will prefer not to have oil used on the skin and talcum powder may be an alternative. Talcum does not provide the same level of lubrication as oil or cream but is particularly suitable for deeper, localised manipulations such as some of those used in sports massage.

Cologne

Cologne is useful to remove excess oil from the skin after the massage, should it be necessary, and to cleanse the soles of the feet before starting massage.

Surgical spirit

Surgical spirit is used to wipe clean any area of the equipment requiring it. For example, it can be used to clean bowls or to clean away any oil spilt on the trolley.

If facial massage is included in your treatments, you will need cleansers to suit the main skin types and products for specialised facial treatments.

When commercial products are used, there should be opportunities for the client to discuss and purchase those suitable for home use. They may be displayed in the cubicle as well as in the reception area.

Progress Check

List the items which should be placed on the trolley before a massage.

Optional extras

Music

Some therapists like to have music playing while working; however, the choice of music is a difficult matter. Many clients will prefer silence and, even if they agree to music, it is unlikely that their choice will coincide with the therapist's, so a selection of music types should be available. The client could be encouraged to bring their favourite tape or disc. If music is played, there should be no attempt to fit the rhythm of the massage to the music. There are recordings made now of special music for relaxation to accompany massage or similar treatments, but again make sure the client is not annoyed by the music.

Refreshment

Clients may be offered some refreshment after the massage and before leaving the salon. Chilled water or fruit juices, coffee, tea or herbal teas are all suitable.

Key Terms

You need to know what these words mean. Go back through the chapter or check in the glossary to find out.

- Decor
- Environment
- Hygiene
- Mineral oil
- Portable
- Temperature
- Patch test

CONSULTATION

3

After working through this chapter you will be able to:

♦ recognise the importance of client consultation

♦ list the components of a client consultation

♦ recognise the need for tact and understanding when carrying out a consultation

♦ recognise the need for a comprehensive client record system

♦ carry out an effective consultation with regard to massage

♦ describe contraindications to body massage

♦ describe conditions requiring special care

♦ recognise conditions requiring medical referral.

Clients may approach a therapist for massage treatments in a number of ways. They may be recommended by another therapist or client or they might contact you as a result of advertising that you have placed. Whatever is the case, an initial consultation must be arranged before treatment is carried out. Information is obtained by questioning and by examining the areas to be treated either as part of the initial consultation or later, during treatment.

> **REMEMBER**
> Consultation is a continuing process.

Aims of a consultation

The aims of a consultation are to:

♦ find out what the client wants from the treatment

♦ determine what the client needs from the treatment

♦ ensure that the client is suitable for treatment

♦ determine any need for special care

♦ establish a good rapport

♦ answer the client's queries

♦ agree a treatment plan.

> **GOOD PRACTICE**
>
> If a treatment or course of treatments is agreed, the client should fully understand the cost and timing of the treatments as no one should be asked to commit themselves to a treatment without fully understanding what is entailed.

Records of consultations and treatments must be kept. A card or computer system should be devised that allows space for answers to all the questions of the consultation and the results of the examination. A typical record card will contain personal and medical details on one side and a record of attendance and treatments on the other.

When asking personal questions it is important that the therapist maintains a courteous and professional manner and explains the importance of a thorough consultation to the client. The client and therapist should be seated comfortably in an area where they cannot be overheard.

Rather than asking a long list of questions related to the health and lifestyle of the client, questions should be phrased occasionally as open questions to allow the client to answer in their own way and express themselves fully. For example, instead of asking, 'Have you ever had diabetes?' you might say, 'What sort of health problems have you had?' A questions that can be answered with a 'yes' or 'no' is a closed questions. A question that cannot be answered with a 'yes' or 'no' is open. Open questions often begin with 'How', 'Why', 'Where', 'What' or 'When'.

GOOD PRACTICE

When carrying out a consultation with elderly or disabled clients, care must be taken to offer help where needed without giving the impression of being patronising or overprotective. (This is a skill that needs a lot of practice!)

Essential information

A consultation card should record essential information about the client.

- Personal details are needed to contact the client, perhaps about altering an appointment or to include in an appropriate future mailshot.
- Medical details are needed to establish the presence or absence of any contraindications to body massage or whether medical referral may be necessary. This also gives the opportunity to discover any conditions requiring special care and to note any localised conditions affecting treatment of that area, for example a past history of low back pain.

This essential information should be arranged on a consultation card (see example on page 17) and clients should be asked to sign to confirm that the information given is correct.

Further questions may be asked, for instance about the client's lifestyle and levels of stress or why the client has chosen to attend for a massage treatment and what they expect from a treatment. These questions will vary between therapists depending on their preference.

A client may have worries or concerns about the nature of the treatment and should be given the opportunity to express these and ask any questions about the treatment.

On the reverse of a consultation card, it is customary to keep a record of attendances, treatments and any reactions to the treatment that are noted at the time or later.

GOOD PRACTICE

Asking clients questions about their health requires tact and sensitivity. It is usually appropriate to explain to the client why it is necessary to ask the questions. Take care to reassure the client that all records are confidential.

SURNAME	FORENAMES ....
ADDRESS	HOME Tel. No. ....
....	WORK Tel. No. ....
DATE of BIRTH	OCCUPATION ....
DATE of FIRST CONSULTATION	
NAME of DOCTOR	TEL. No. ....
GENERAL STATE OF HEALTH	
....	
CURRENT MEDICATION	
CURRENT MEDICAL TREATMENT	
CURRENT ALTERNATIVE/COMPLEMENTARY TREATMENTS	
....	
PAST MEDICAL/SURGICAL HISTORY with APPROXIMATE DATES	
....	
CLIENT SIGNATURE .... DATE	

Figure 3.1 *An example of a consultation card*

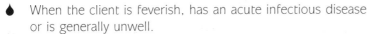

There are few complete contraindications to a full body massage but there are many localised ones. With some contraindications it may be advisable to consult the client's doctor.

Contraindications
to any massage

- When the client is feverish, has an acute infectious disease or is generally unwell.
- During the active phase of rheumatoid arthritis.
- When the client is being treated for cancer, unless the massage is carried out under medical supervision.
- When the client is under the influence of drink or drugs.
- If the client is pregnant and you have reason to believe that the pregnancy is unstable.

REMEMBER
'Contraindication' means that the treatment should not be given.

Contraindications
to localised massage

- Over a limb where there is a history of thrombosis or phlebitis in the blood vessels.
- Over an area of a skin disorder which may be spread.
- Over an area of inflammation such as a rash or boil.
- Over an area of sunburn.
- Over bruising, cuts, recent scars or abrasions or very thin, fragile skin.
- Over recent sprains, fractures or surgical procedures.
- Over a joint that is hot or swollen.

- Over any area of swelling.
- Over very tender or painful muscles.
- Directly over severe varicose veins.
- Directly over moles and warts.
- Over the abdomen during early (first three months) of pregnancy. Very gentle stroking movements may be used in later stages.

REMEMBER

A doctor will not release any information about a patient unless the patient has given the doctor permission in writing.

If a client is on any long-term medication then it may be necessary to contact the client's doctor for advice, with the permission of the client.

Conditions where special care should be exercised
Diabetes
In some diabetics, circulation is poor, skin sensation may be altered and the skin can become very fragile. The healing process can be very slow – this is especially a problem in the lower leg and foot.

Epilepsy
Most people with epilepsy have their condition well controlled with medication but special care must be taken not to leave them unattended on a couch.

Heart disease or blood pressure disorders
Very often a client with these conditions will benefit from massage but the client may need special care. Someone with high blood pressure or heart disease may need to avoid lying flat, whereas someone with low blood pressure may feel faint on sitting up and require support. Patients with heart problems should not be massaged over the front of the chest or neck.

When a consultation has been completed, you should check that there are no contraindications to treatment. The client's signature that the information given is correct is a safeguard for the therapist. This is often a convenient time to agree appointment times and confirm the cost of the treatment. The client should be given the opportunity to ask any questions related to the treatment or the consultation.

Client records must be kept safely in a secure place and updated whenever the client attends for treatment. A full record of treatments given, products used and any special requirements needed should be kept and referred to. If records are kept on computer then the Data Protection Act applies and the therapist should conform to the requirements of the act.

Data Protection Act
The Data Protection Act gives clients the right to see personal data held on computer about them and to get it corrected if it is wrong. Computer users who keep information about individuals must, by law, appear in the Data Protection Register.

ACTIVITY

Working with a partner, role-play a consultation with a new client. Imagine that the client has never had massage before but has been recommended to you by another client. Ask a colleague to watch the role-play and give feedback on how successful you were in putting the client at ease and eliciting the correct information.

Key Terms

You need to know what these words mean. Go back through the chapter or check in the glossary to find out.

- Closed questions
- Contraindications
- Medical details
- Medication
- Open questions
- Personal details
- Rapport

After working through this chapter you will be able to:

- describe the main features of the body systems relevant to body massage
- describe the main functions of these systems
- describe the main effects of massage on these body systems
- relate any contraindications of massage to these systems and their structure and function
- describe the effects of stress on the body
- relate the effects of massage to the management of stress
- relate any specific effects of aromatherapy massage on these systems.

The systems of the body relevant to body massage

a) Integumentary system (skin and its derivatives such as nails and hair).
b) Musculo-skeletal system (bones, joints and muscles).
c) Circulatory system.
d) Lymphatic system.
e) Nervous system.
f) Respiratory system.
g) Digestive system.
h) Renal system.
i) Endocrine system.
j) Immune system.

Integumentary system

The integumentary system is the name given to the skin and its derivatives (hair, nails and glands). The skin is the part of the integumentary system which forms the outer surface of the body and is the part of the body which is immediately affected by massage. The skin envelopes the body and is the largest organ in the body, covering on an adult an area of approximately two square metres. Skin varies in thickness in different parts of the body from very thin skin, about 0.10 mm thick, on the eyelids and lips to much thicker skin on the soles of the feet or palms of the hands, which is approximately 3.5 mm at its thickest.

Structure

The skin is composed of two main layers – the epidermis and the deeper dermis. The epidermis itself consists of five layers, each called a stratum.

Stratum corneum

This is the superficial layer. It is made of many rows of flattened, dead cells which contain the tough protein keratin. The outer cells of this layer are shed regularly and some of them will be rubbed off by massage, especially if a body-peeling cream is used to prepare the skin for massage.

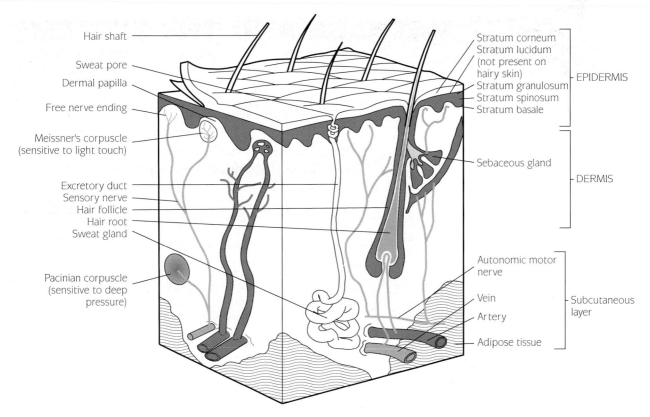

Figure 4.1 *Sectional view of the skin*

Stratum lucidum

This is a clear layer formed by three or four rows of clear, flat, dead cells and is found only in the palms of the hands and soles of the feet where it acts to resist friction.

Stratum granulosum

This is a layer of two or three rows of cells which contain a substance involved in the formation of keratin.

Stratum spinosum

This is a layer of eight to ten rows of many-sided cells fitting closely together. The stratum spinosum together with the deepest layer of the epidermis helps to form new cells.

Stratum basale

This deepest layer of the epidermis is a single row of oblong, columnar cells that divide continually. As the cells of the stratum basale multiply, they push up to the surface, progressively becoming part of the upper layers of the epidermis until they die and are shed from the stratum corneum. In this way, the epidermis is replaced regularly every few weeks.

The dermis is the deeper layer of the skin and it is much thicker than the epidermis. It contains the connective tissue, which gives the skin its elasticity and strength, as well as hair follicles, blood vessels, nerves and glands.

The upper part of the dermis has finger-like projections that extend into the epidermis. This papillary layer of the dermis contains nerve endings which are sensitive to touch. Some called Meissner's corpuscles sense light touch while others called Pacinian corpuscles are sensitive to deep pressure, so it is here that the difference between various massage movements are registered.

The dermis also contains blood and lymph vessels, nerves, hair follicles, sweat glands and collagenous and elastic connective tissue fibres.

The elastic connective tissues become less efficient during the ageing process. It is this loss of elasticity which explains why the skin of older people is looser and more wrinkled. This laxity of the skin is one of the factors that must be taken into account when massaging an older client as too deep or brisk effleurage movements could be very uncomfortable.

ACTIVITY

Pinch the skin on the back of your hand, release it and note how long it takes to return to normal. Ask a number of people of different ages to do the same and note the differences.

Hair grows from a root deep in the dermis. The shaft of the hair passes through the epidermis to project above the surface of the skin. It is present on most of the body areas covered by massage except the soles of the feet and palms of the hands. Hair varies in length and texture in different parts of the body. In its usual position, hair lies at an angle to the skin and where possible massage strokes should be in the direction of this natural lie of the hair, especially if the hair is long or very vigorous.

The dermis contains the blood vessels that supply the skin. These capillaries dilate or constrict in response to external factors – mainly heat and cold. When the capillaries are dilated, more blood flows close to the surface of the skin and when they are constricted less blood flows. Depending on the amount of pigment in the skin, the dilation and constriction of capillaries in the dermis may affect the skin colour temporarily. Warm skin looks redder than cool skin. This will be noted in massage treatments as the massage warms the skin. The reddening is called an erythema.

Lymph capillaries are blind-ended tubes that begin in spaces between cells and are present in the deeper part of the skin. More mention is made of these in the section on the lymphatic system (page 37).

There are two types of glands present in the dermis which have openings to the surface of the skin. These are the sweat glands and the sebaceous glands.

Sweat glands are found over the surface of the body and are most numerous on the soles of the feet and the palms of the hands. They are also very numerous on the forehead and armpits. Each gland has a coiled part in the dermis and a tube leading to a pore on the surface. They produce a thin watery salty fluid, commonly known as perspiration or sweat. Their main function is to regulate body temperature by producing sweat in response to heat. The body cools as the sweat evaporates. A client who becomes very warm during a massage may sweat excessively and this may result in the therapist's hands slipping too much. It is also possible that the therapist's hands may sweat too much with the same result. Excessive sweating on the palms of the hands can occur if the therapist is nervous for any reason and is often a problem for a student. With time and confidence the problem diminishes.

The second type of gland is the sebaceous gland. These glands are situated in the hair follicles and produce an oily liquid called sebum. Sebaceous glands are not found on the soles of the feet or palms of the hand and are quite small in the skin covering most of the trunk and limbs. They are large on the upper chest, face and neck. The sebum produced by the glands keeps the skin and hair soft and supple. The production of sebum is often stimulated by massage. Beneath the dermis is a layer of connective tissue containing adipose tissue.

Adipose tissue

This is a type of loose connective tissue containing cells which are specially adapted to store fat. Adipose tissue is found under the skin and around organs. It acts as a reserve of food and as it is a poor conductor of heat, helps to maintain body temperature by preventing heat loss.

Massage is often said to affect adipose tissue by softening hard fat under the skin and helping it to disperse into the deeper tissue and circulatory system. Many massage creams are also said to help with the dispersal of subcutaneous fat.

The distribution of the fat layer under the skin varies according to sex, age and lifestyle. Women tend to have a thicker layer of adipose tissue than men giving the female body a softer outline with the muscles being less obvious. After the menopause, women tend to put on weight in the more masculine pattern i.e. on the waist and abdomen rather than the hips and thighs.

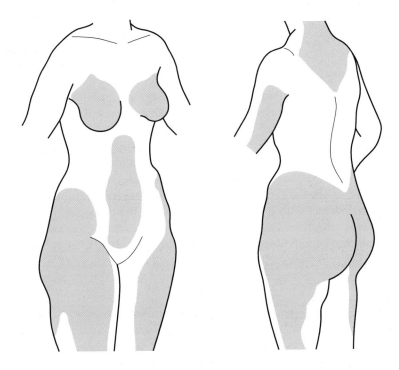

Figure 4.2 *Fat distribution (female)*

Absorption

For many years, biologists thought that the skin formed an impervious barrier to external substances, but more recent research shows that most chemicals placed on the skin can be absorbed to some degree despite the skin's protective mechanisms. Some chemicals are absorbed only into the skin and some penetrate across the skin to enter the bloodstream and travel around the body. In some cases this effect can be beneficial. For example, drugs for the treatment of heart and endocrine disorders can be delivered by means of patches containing the drugs being placed on the skin. In other cases the absorption of chemicals through the skin may be very harmful, which is why industrial workers handling hazardous materials such as mercury or pesticides will wear protective clothing.

There are many factors which determine how much of a chemical penetrates the skin. Some of these factors are:

- the amount and concentration of the chemical applied
- the length of time the chemical is in contact with the skin
- the skin's temperature and moisture content
- the concentration of hair follicles and sweat ducts in the area where the chemical is applied
- whether the skin is damaged in any way.

All of these are likely to affect the absorption of substances used in massage. They are particularly relevant to the application of essential oils used in aromatherapy.

Research on the absorption of essential oils has shown that they pass through the epidermis and enter the lymphatic and blood vessels in the dermis. In work done to research the skin penetration of fragrance chemicals, it has been shown that absorption is greater over areas of thinner more delicate skin such as that on the face and eyelids and less on the thicker skin of the legs, trunk and abdomen. Children's skin is more permeable than adults'.

The two major factors governing the level of absorption of such chemicals by the skin appear to be the strength of the dose applied and the size of the area to which it is applied. Massage and heat may also encourage absorption as will covering the area with clothes or towels.

Allergy

Substances applied to the skin may cause the skin to react allergically against the substance. The reaction of some of the cells of the dermis is to release histamine causing the tissue to become red, warm and swollen. The first contact with the substance may leave the tissue sensitised so that later contact can cause a more severe and generalised reaction. Once a person has become sensitised to a substance it must be completely avoided.

SAFE PRACTICE

Clients should always be asked if they are allergic to any substances used in products being applied to the skin. If there is any doubt, perform a patch test. Apply some of the substance to a small patch of skin and check for any reaction 24 hours later.

Aromatherapy products which contain the essential oils of plants are often considered safe because they are pure and natural. However, they are potent, concentrated, natural chemicals and some can be toxic. For example, the oil from the pennyroyal plant contains a liver toxin and cinnamon bark oil can cause allergic skin reactions. The contraindications of individual oils must be checked before use on the skin. The commonest way of applying these essential oils is by massage which increases the flow of blood to the area and this may enhance absorption of the substances into the body.

Photosensitivity

Certain chemicals cause the skin to react more strongly than usual when exposed to sunlight. Care needs to be taken with citrus essential oils which are obtained from the peel of the fruit and which contain furo-coumarin molecules. The best known of these is oil of bergamot, used in perfumery and aromatherapy. The result can be 'sunburn' or a rash after a very short exposure to ultraviolet light.

GOOD PRACTICE

Any product containing a photosensitiser should not be applied to the skin before exposure to natural or artificial sunlight (for example, a sunbed.)

Effects of massage on skin

- Desquamation – the removal of dead cells from the surface, improving skin texture.
- Stimulation of sweat and sebaceous glands giving a 'cleansing' effect.
- Improving the circulation to the skin, increasing nourishment and assisting the removal of waste products.
- Warming the skin temporarily producing an erythema.

Products used on the skin during massage will have their own specific effects.

Contraindications
to massage over a particular area of skin

- any skin infection
- any area of very thin fragile skin
- severe bruising
- breaks in the skin
- moles and warts
- sunburn
- any contraindication to specific products used.

Key Terms

You need to know what these words mean. Go back through the chapter or check in the glossary to find out.

- Adipose tissue
- Allergy

- Collagen
- Connective tissue
- Dermis
- Desquamation
- Epidermis
- Erythema
- Histamine
- Keratin
- Patch test

The musculo-skeletal system

The skeleton is constructed from dense connective tissue as are the ligaments which attach bone to bone at the joints and the tendons which attach muscle to bone. Massage over tendons and ligaments can help to keep them flexible and is of particular value in a sports massage.

Massage is unlikely to have a direct effect on the bony skeleton or the joints, but may have an indirect effect through stimulating the blood supply. It is important for therapists to know the position of the parts of the skeleton and recognise those superficial areas which protrude in some clients and which require special care during massage. During a sports massage, knowledge of the whole musculo-skeletal system is of great importance. In a sports massage, the massage is often aimed at specific problem areas with the massage strokes following the direction of the muscle fibres or being directed across them depending on the effects required.

The skeleton

The skeleton forms the framework of the body and is formed of bone and cartilage. Bones are attached to each other at joints where they are held together by ligaments and muscles.

Functions of the skeleton

The skeleton:

- supports the soft tissues of the body
- protects structures such as the brain, spinal cord and heart
- stores salts such as calcium
- produces blood cells in the marrow of the bone.

Structure of the skeleton

The skeleton is made up of 206 bones. It is divided into two main parts, the axial skeleton and the appendicular skeleton.

The axial skeleton is made up of bones which lie around the centre of the body. The bones of the axial skeleton are listed in Table 4.1 (page 27).

The appendicular skeleton consists of the bones of the upper and lower limbs and the bones that attach them to the axial skeleton, the pectoral girdle and the pelvic girdle. The bones of the appendicular skeleton are listed in Table 4.2 (page 27).

In massage, the outline of the skeleton is followed and bony points that are not covered by soft tissue must be treated lightly. Some points can be

	Bones	Number of bones
Head	Cranium	8
	Face	14
	Ear	6
	Hyoid (in throat)	1
Thorax	Sternum	1
	Ribs	24
Spine	Vertebrae	26

Table 4.1 *Bones of the axial skeleton*

Components		Number of bones
Pectoral girdle	Clavicle	2
	Scapula	2
Upper limbs		60
Pelvic girdle	Pelvic bones	2
Lower limbs		60

Table 4.2 *Bones of the appendicular skeleton*

very painful if deep movements are applied. As the hands are very sensitive, the difference between soft tissue such as fat or muscle and hard bony tissue should be easily felt and massage to the obvious bony points should be avoided.

Contraindications

to massage and points of special care related to the skeleton

- Massage should not be applied over a fractured bone until it is completely healed.
- If metal plates and pins have been inserted in the bones, care must be taken over the area and medical advice sought.
- Any condition under medical care.
- Any unexplained bone pain.

ACTIVITY

Find the following prominent bony points on Figures 4.3 and 4.4 (page 28) and on yourself from the head down.

- Base of the occipital bone.
- Mastoid process.
- 7th cervical vertebra.
- Clavicle.
- Spine of the scapula.
- Acromion process.
- Olecranon process (take care here: a nerve crosses the elbow – commonly called the funny bone).
- Styloid process of the ulna.

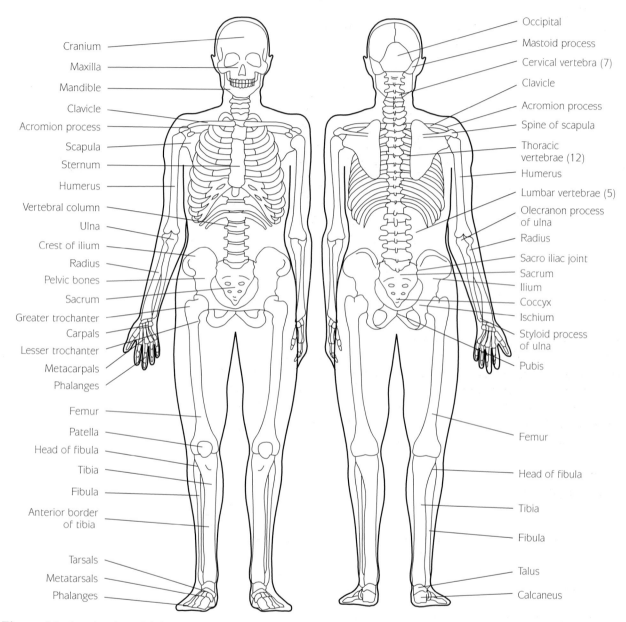

- Crest of the Ilium.
- Sacro-Iliac joint.
- Greater trochanter of the femur.
- Patella.
- Anterior border of the tibia.
- Head of the fibula (take care, another nerve crosses here).

Labels on left figure (anterior view):
Cranium
Maxilla
Mandible
Clavicle
Acromion process
Scapula
Sternum
Humerus
Vertebral column
Ulna
Crest of ilium
Radius
Pelvic bones
Sacrum
Greater trochanter
Carpals
Lesser trochanter
Metacarpals
Phalanges
Femur
Patella
Head of fibula
Tibia
Fibula
Anterior border of tibia
Tarsals
Metatarsals
Phalanges

Labels on right figure (posterior view):
Occipital
Mastoid process
Cervical vertebra (7)
Clavicle
Acromion process
Spine of scapula
Thoracic vertebrae (12)
Humerus
Lumbar vertebrae (5)
Olecranon process of ulna
Radius
Sacro iliac joint
Sacrum
Ilium
Coccyx
Ischium
Styloid process of ulna
Pubis
Femur
Head of fibula
Tibia
Fibula
Talus
Calcaneus

Figure 4.3 *Anterior view of skeleton*

Figure 4.4 *Posterior view of skeleton*

Joints

A joint is a place where bones in the body meet. At some joints such as those of the adult skull, the bones interlock so that there is no movement between them. At other joints such as those formed between the bodies of the vertebrae, the bones are loosely connected by flexible cartilage which allows only limited movement. A third kind of joint allows free movement between the bones. This kind of joint is known as a synovial joint.

Synovial joints are the most numerous type of joint in the body. They have a number of common features.

- Muscles surround the joint.
- Ligaments hold the bones together.
- A capsule of connective tissue encloses the joint.
- A synovial membrane lines the capsule.
- Synovial fluid is produced by the synovial membrane to lubricate the joint.
- Cartilage covers the bony surfaces where they meet.

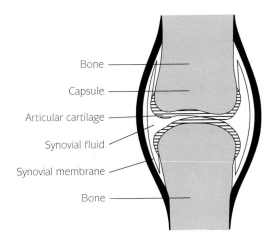

Figure 4.5 *Section through a synovial joint*

Massage affects the joints indirectly by stimulating the circulation and lymphatic flow in the region of the joint. Some therapists may include a series of passive movements in a massage treatment. A passive movement is one where the therapist moves a joint through a range of movements while the client is relaxed. They are thought to improve the mobility of the joints and aid the circulation. Passive movements are often included in a shiatsu massage.

Contraindications

to massage related to the joints

- Over any swelling of a joint when the cause is not known.
- Over any joint that is hot or painful.
- Over any joint where a strain or sprain is suspected.

ACTIVITY

Find out as much as possible about various forms of arthritis, for example rheumatoid arthritis, osteoarthritis and ankylosing spondylitis. Also find out if there are any other conditions which might limit movement in synovial joints.

Muscle tissue

There are three types of muscle tissue: skeletal, cardiac and visceral. Skeletal muscle tissue forms the muscles that are felt during massage. Muscle tissue makes up 40–50 % of body weight.

- It is excitable in that it receives and responds to stimuli by way of nerve impulses.
- It can contract, shortening and thickening when stimulated.
- It can be stretched.
- It is elastic, returning to its original shape after contracting or being stretched.

Skeletal (voluntary) muscle is attached to bones by means of connective tissue such as tendons and, as its name suggests, it is under voluntary control. For a muscle fibre to contract it must first be stimulated by a nerve cell.

Individual muscles or groups of muscle fibres have their own nerve and blood supplies. Muscle contraction requires a good blood supply to bring oxygen and nutrients to provide energy and to remove the waste products of contraction. By contracting, skeletal muscles perform three important functions. They:

- move parts of the body
- maintain the upright posture of the body
- produce heat – a by-product of work done by the muscle in contracting.

Some massage movements, particularly tapotement movements such as hacking, can cause muscle fibres to contract. This repetitive contraction and relaxation of the muscle fibres stimulates blood flow in the same way that exercise does. Hacking has been shown to be much more effective than any other massage stroke in increasing blood flow to muscles.

Muscles tend to work in groups and when one group of muscles works to produce a movement there will be an opposing group of muscles which has to relax to allow the movement to happen. For example the muscles in front of the upper arm (biceps and brachialis) contract to bend the elbow, but the elbow would not be able to move unless the muscles on the back of the arm (triceps) relax.

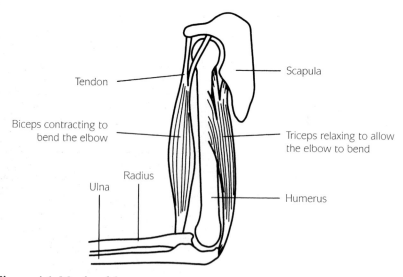

Figure 4.6 *Muscles of the upper arm*

Muscle tone

At any given time, some fibres in a muscle are contracted while others are relaxed. Not enough fibres are contracted to produce movement, but this helps to maintain posture without any noticeable effort. This partial muscle contraction is called muscle tone and the term is commonly used to describe the firmness or flabbiness of muscle. Good muscle tone is achieved and maintained by exercise but some massage movements, such as hacking, that stretch muscle fibres may help to maintain the tone of superficial muscles. Massage is adapted to suit clients with different levels of muscle tone so that the massage used on an elderly client who exercises infrequently will be very different from that used on a sportsman or sportswoman who has firm well-toned muscles. It is important that a therapist's hands develop sensitivity to these differences.

Muscle fatigue

During gentle or moderate exercise, muscles are able to obtain sufficient energy by oxidising glucose in the body. As exercise increases, there is not enough oxygen available and energy is produced from glucose anaerobically. A waste product called lactic acid is produced when muscles produce energy anaerobically. Lactic acid builds up in the muscles slowing them down and sometimes causing cramp. One of the purposes of massage after exercise is to aid the removal of lactic acid from the muscles.

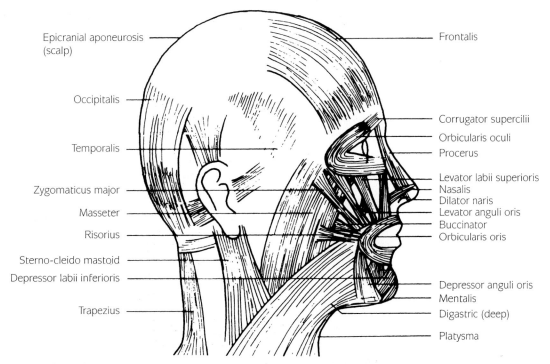

Figure 4.7 *Facial muscles*

Massage is often used to relax muscles, either by general massage to bring about relaxation of the whole body or by working on specific muscles, such as those used in particular movements. In either case a knowledge of the shape and position of the superficial muscles of the body is important. In sports massage in particular, the massage strokes will be directed along the length of muscle fibres or across them depending on the effects required.

Some muscles are small and delicate such as the muscles of the face, and here in particular massage movements should follow the direction of the muscle fibres where possible.

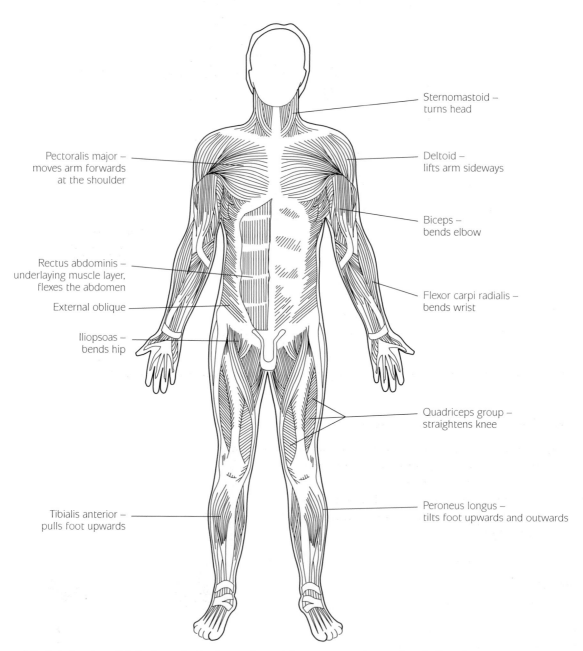

Sternomastoid – turns head

Pectoralis major – moves arm forwards at the shoulder

Deltoid – lifts arm sideways

Biceps – bends elbow

Rectus abdominis – underlaying muscle layer, flexes the abdomen

External oblique

Iliopsoas – bends hip

Flexor carpi radialis – bends wrist

Quadriceps group – straightens knee

Peroneus longus – tilts foot upwards and outwards

Tibialis anterior – pulls foot upwards

Figure 4.8 *Anterior view of skeletal muscles (main muscles and the movements they perform indicated)*

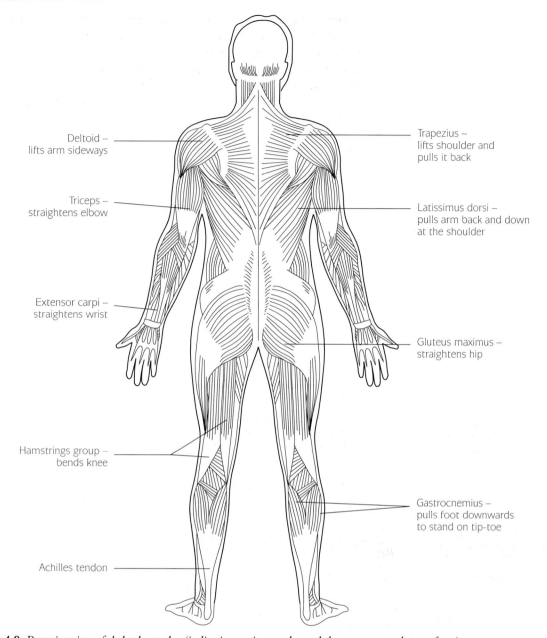

Deltoid –
lifts arm sideways

Triceps –
straightens elbow

Extensor carpi –
straightens wrist

Hamstrings group –
bends knee

Achilles tendon

Trapezius –
lifts shoulder and
pulls it back

Latissimus dorsi –
pulls arm back and down
at the shoulder

Gluteus maximus –
straightens hip

Gastrocnemius –
pulls foot downwards
to stand on tip-toe

Figure 4.9 *Posterior view of skeletal muscles (indicating main muscles and the movements they perform)*

Effects of massage on muscle tissue

- Stimulates the blood supply which brings fresh nutrients and oxygen to the muscles and removes waste products.
- Helps to reduce muscle fatigue.
- Helps to maintain the elasticity of muscle fibres.
- Helps to reduce adhesions in muscle which may have developed following injury.

Contraindications

to massage related to the muscles

- Over muscles which are painful.
- Over muscles which are tender.

The circulatory system

Blood is a complex fluid consisting of a variety of red and white blood cells, platelets and the liquid plasma. The functions of blood are to:

- transport oxygen from the lungs to the cells of the body
- transport carbon dioxide from the cells to the lungs
- transport nutrients from the digestive organs to the cells
- transport waste products from the cells to the kidneys, lungs and sweat glands
- transport hormones from the endocrine glands to the cells
- transport enzymes to various cells
- regulate the pH of the body
- help to regulate body temperature
- regulate the water content of cells
- protect the body against infection and toxic substances.

The heart is the centre of the cardiovascular system. It is a hollow, muscular organ about the size of a clenched fist. It is located in the centre of the chest between the lungs and is tilted to the left. Its function is to pump blood through the blood vessels of the body. It acts as a double pump, the right side pumps deoxygenated blood to the lungs to receive oxygen while the left side pumps oxygenated blood from the lungs to the rest of the body.

Blood is carried around the body in blood vessels. These are:

- arteries – which carry blood from the heart
- veins – which carry blood to the heart
- capillaries – which link arteries to veins.

The heart pumps oxygenated blood into large arteries which then branch into smaller and smaller arteries. The smallest of these arteries are called arterioles and they reach to all parts of the body. The arterioles link with the tiny capillaries in the tissues which in turn connect with the smallest veins, called venules. Venules join up to form veins which return the blood to the heart.

Arteries and veins differ in structure. Arteries have thicker walls which contain muscle fibres to help control the flow of blood through them. Every time the heart beats, it pushes blood through the arteries and it can be felt in large arteries as the pulse, for example the radial pulse at the wrist.

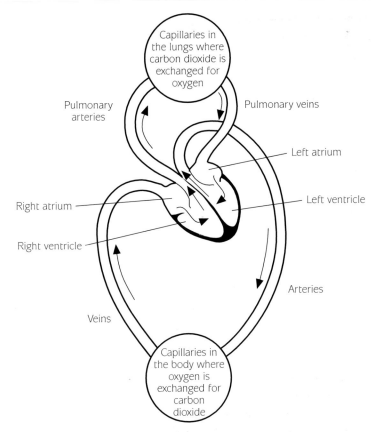

Figure 4.10 *The double circulatory system of the body*

Veins have thinner walls than arteries and some veins have valves to prevent the blood flowing backwards. Blood is kept moving in veins by the squeezing action of surrounding muscles contracting and relaxing and to a lesser degree by the pressure in the arteries pushing blood through the capillaries and veins.

Varicose veins is a condition where the valves fail to keep the blood from flowing backwards and the walls of the veins bulge, becoming very prominent. They are often caused by standing for long periods without sufficient muscular activity and also occur in some women in pregnancy. The skin over the region of severe varicose veins is often thin and papery and if damaged may break down to form ulcers.

GOOD PRACTICE

Care must always be taken when working over an area of fragile skin.

Occasionally, clots may form in the blood in places that cause problems. Examples of this are the clots which can form in the arteries of the heart muscle (coronary arteries) which can cause a heart attack, and the clots which can form in the arteries to the brain which can cause strokes.

Clots may also form in veins, particularly in the legs in both superficial and deep veins. When clots are formed in superficial veins, the condition is called thrombophlebitis and is often associated with varicose veins. The area is usually warm, swollen and is very tender and painful.

When a clot, or thrombus, forms in a deep vein the condition is called deep venous thrombosis. This condition may follow surgery, hormonal treatment or travel in cramped conditions, such as a long air flight where movement of the legs is limited. There will be localised swelling in the limb affected but there is often no pain unless the area is probed quite deeply.

SAFE PRACTICE

Neither thrombophlebitis nor deep venous thrombosis should ever be treated by massage. Localised swelling, especially in the calf of one leg should always be referred to a doctor. If massage is carried out there is a risk that the clot may be moved on or broken up. The clot, or fragments of it, may then travel through the circulatory system to the lungs where they may cause great harm. If the client has had either of these conditions in the past then clearance should be sought from the client's doctor before treating the area.

Massage strokes such as effleurage can help the return of blood through the veins as the strokes are performed in the direction of venous flow towards the heart.

ACTIVITY

Firmly stroke the inside of your arm upwards from wrist to elbow. Note the emptying of the superficial veins followed by rapid filling.

Blood pressure

The pressure of the blood in the arteries and arterioles reaches a peak when the heart contracts; this is called the systolic blood pressure. It gradually decreases to the minimum allowed by the elasticity of the artery walls, the diastolic blood pressure, just before the next contraction. Blood pressure is always recorded in two figures, the systolic pressure being shown over the diastolic pressure, for example 120/80. The figures represent the pressures measured in millimetres of mercury.

Blood pressure varies with age, sex and weight. It tends to increase with age. It may be raised for short periods by exercise or stress and anxiety and be lowered by rest and contentment.

High blood pressure

When people have a blood pressure that is at a continuously high level they will be at a greater risk of strokes, heart attacks and kidney damage. Consequently many clients with high blood pressure will be taking medication to modify it. Clients with high blood pressure may be more comfortable if they do not lie completely flat during treatment.

Low blood pressure

Blood pressure must be sufficient to pump blood to the brain when the body is in the upright position If it is not, then the person will faint. Some people with low blood pressure may feel faint when sitting up suddenly from the lying position.

Effects of massage on the circulatory system

◆ Speeds the flow of blood through the veins.
◆ Causes dilation of superficial capillaries producing skin erythema.

- Stimulates the supply of fresh, oxygenated blood to the superficial tissues.
- Stimulates the removal of waste products from the superficial tissues.
- Reduces the viscosity, or stickiness of the blood.
- May reduce blood pressure probably due to psychological factors.

Contraindications

to massage related to the circulatory system

- Over an area which has, or has had in the past, a deep venous thrombosis or thrombophlebitis.
- Over obvious varicose veins.
- Over an area of swelling or tenderness.

ACTIVITY

Find out what the 'normal' range of blood pressure is.

Key Terms

You need to know what these words mean. Go back through the section or check in the glossary to find out.

- Arterioles
- Capillaries
- Enzymes
- Hormones
- pH value
- Thrombus
- Toxic
- Venule

The lymphatic system

The lymphatic system supplements the circulatory system by removing excess fluid from the tissues. It consists of:

- lymph nodes, often called lymph glands, which are linked together by
- lymph vessels and capillaries (large and small thin-walled tubes scattered through the tissues of the body)
- lymphatic tissue, found in associated organs such as the tonsils, adenoids, spleen and liver.

The lymphatic capillaries collect excess fluid from the body along with any bacteria, viruses and other particles that need removing from the tissues. This fluid is called lymph and passes through the capillaries which join to form larger lymphatic vessels. The lymph passes through lymph nodes where the unwanted particles are filtered out and removed. Eventually the vessels join to become two large vessels that empty their contents back into the main circulatory system at the veins in the base of the neck.

The functions of the lymphatic system are to:

♦ remove excess fluid from the tissues
♦ filter out unwanted material
♦ help to absorb fat from around the intestine
♦ transport fats and fat soluble vitamins
♦ produce T-lymphocytes and B-lymphocytes, which destroy bacteria and viruses
♦ produce antibodies as part of the body's immune system.

Lymph nodes sometimes swell when there is an infection in the locality because the nodes make large quantities of lymphocytes with which to fight infection. Thus the nodes of the neck can swell when there is a throat infection. Infection can also travel along lymphatic vessels until a group of nodes is reached. For example, if a hand is infected, the nodes in the elbow or armpit may swell. Other matter, such as cancer cells, may be spread along the lymphatic pathways, therefore surgery or radiotherapy for localised cancer may be targeted at particular lymph nodes.

A condition called lymphoedema may occur following such treatment for cancer. Lymphoedema is a condition where the lymphatic drainage is no longer effective in draining the limb concerned. The limb affected will be very swollen and hard. Massage to a limb affected by lymphoedema should only be given by a therapist fully trained in manual lymph drainage techniques. Deep Swedish-style massage may cause more harm than good.

More commonly, sluggish lymphatic drainage in part of the system will lead to puffiness often called water retention. The feet and ankles may be swollen in the evening and some people will be uncomfortable in tight clothes as the day passes.

Effects of massage on the lymphatic system

♦ Stimulates the flow of lymph in the lymphatic capillaries and superficial vessels.
♦ Reduces generalised swelling or fluid retention in the tissues.
♦ Stimulates the absorption of waste matter.

Contraindications
to massage related to the lymphatic system

♦ Over swollen lymph nodes.
♦ Over an infected vessel (seen as a red line under the skin leading to swollen nodes).
♦ Cancer, unless under medical supervision.

Massage is often carried out specifically to stimulate superficial lymphatic drainage of part of, or the whole body. When this is the case, strokes will be in the direction of lymphatic drainage towards the nearest lymph nodes.

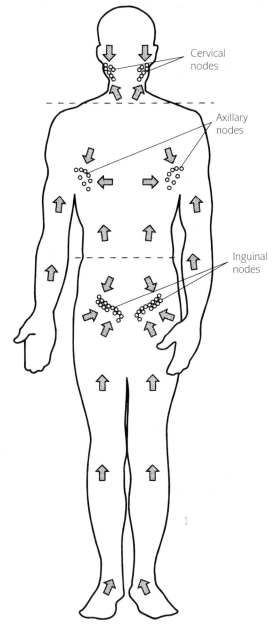

Figure 4.11 *Anterior view of superficial drainage in the lymphatic system*

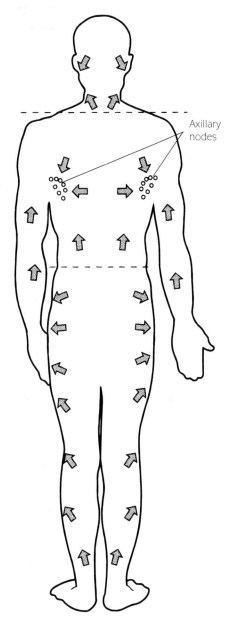

Figure 4.12 *Posterior view of superficial drainage in the lymphatic system*

Key Terms

You need to know what these words mean. Go back through the chapter or check in the glossary to find out.

- Lymph
- Lymph nodes
- Lymphocytes
- Lymphoedema
- Water retention

The nervous system

The function of the nervous system is to carry messages around the body, controlling and co-ordinating other systems. It stimulates movement and together with the endocrine system it maintains homeostasis. It senses change inside and outside the body, interprets those changes and initiates actions to deal with them.

The nervous system consists of:

- the central nervous system which is the control centre – the brain and spinal cord
- the peripheral nervous system – the nerves which carry messages to and from the central nervous system.

All sensations from the body will be relayed by the peripheral nervous system to the central nervous system to be interpreted and acted upon.

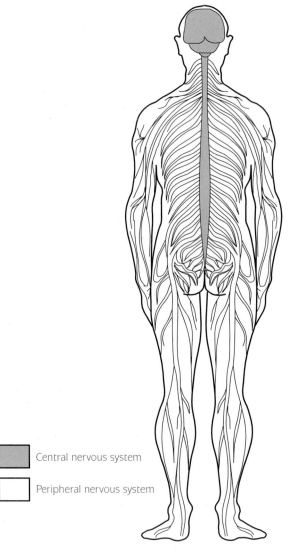

Figure 4.13 *Central and peripheral nervous systems*

The nerves which carry messages from the central nervous system may go to the skeletal muscles to produce movement which is under voluntary control or to involuntary muscle, cardiac muscle and to glands.

This latter part is called the autonomic nervous system and operates without conscious control.

Sensations

A stimulus of some kind will be sensed by a sense organ or receptor and converted into nerve impulses which are conveyed to the sensory part of the brain. The stimulus may be light, heat, smell, or touch and pressure as in the case of massage.

The receptors or sense organs are parts of the body that contain cells that are sensitive to stimuli, for example cells in the eyes, ears, nose and skin.

Receptors called exteroceptors are sensitive to stimuli outside the body and transmit sensations of hearing, sight, smell, touch, pressure, temperature and pain. These exteroceptors are located near the surface of the body. Receptors called interoceptors are sensitive to stimuli originating inside the body such as pain, pressure, taste, fatigue, hunger and thirst. Interoceptors are situated deeper in the body. Receptors called proprioceptors are situated in muscles, tendons and joints and in the inner ear and are sensitive to the position of parts of the body.

When a stimulus is applied continuously, its effect becomes less with time. This is especially true of touch sensations, for example, when you put on your clothes you are aware of them, but the sensation gradually fades. This is called sensory adaptation and has an important role in massage as the client will gradually become accustomed to the feeling of being massaged and be able to relax as this adaptation takes place.

The most obvious sensations relating to massage are those received by receptors in the skin and the connective tissue just under the skin. These receptors are found all over the body, but are denser in some parts than others. Areas with many receptors will be much more sensitive than areas with fewer receptors.

Skin receptors for fine touch are found in the superficial part of the dermis and include Meissner's corpuscles which are most numerous in the fingertips, palms of the hands and soles of the feet. Receptors for deep pressure are deep in the dermis and are called Pacinian corpuscles, they are less sensitive to variations than the fine touch receptors.

The receptors in the skin are important to the therapist and the client. Too light a touch can be very irritating to a client who needs a deep massage and similarly too deep pressure can be painful. The therapist should use the very sensitive palms of the hands to register the reaction of the client which would probably be to tense the muscles in response to discomfort. The massage can then be adapted accordingly.

The autonomic nervous system carries messages from the central nervous system to control and regulate the circulation, breathing, digestion, excretion and the endocrine system. It is divided into two parts which act in different ways to balance each other.

The sympathetic division of the autonomic nervous system prepares the body for action by increasing the heart and respiration rate and increasing blood pressure. More blood will flow to the muscles and less to other areas, digestion is reduced, the skin will feel cold and damp and the

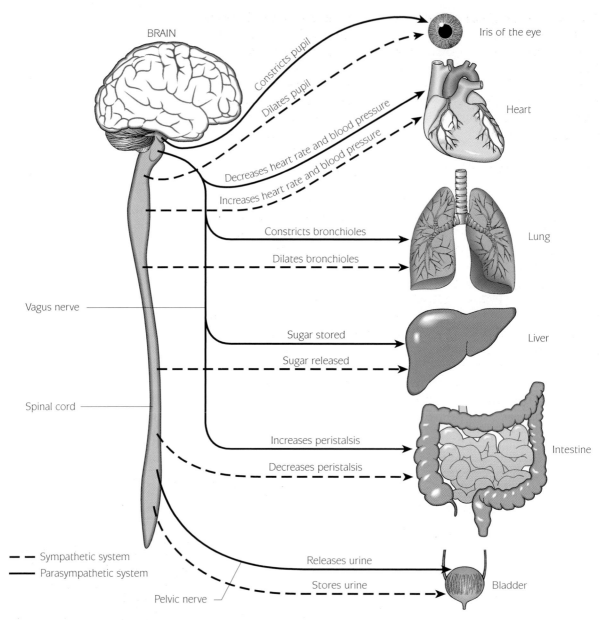

BRAIN

Constricts pupil

Dilates pupil

Iris of the eye

Decreases heart rate and blood pressure

Increases heart rate and blood pressure

Heart

Constricts bronchioles

Dilates bronchioles

Lung

Vagus nerve

Sugar stored

Sugar released

Liver

Spinal cord

Increases peristalsis

Decreases peristalsis

Intestine

– – – Sympathetic system
——— Parasympathetic system

Releases urine

Stores urine

Bladder

Pelvic nerve

Figure 4.14 *Autonomic nervous system*

muscles tense. This may be in response to pain or fear or feelings of stress. The parasympathetic division prepares the body for rest, it decreases heart rate and blood pressure and promotes digestion.

Massage by its nature should bring about relaxation and a reduction of stress. Stress is a necessary part of life that becomes harmful only when it is excessive or continuous to the point where it is difficult to cope with. Too much stress can bring about physical symptoms such as breathlessness, anxiety, tension headaches and insomnia. There are many relaxation techniques such as yoga and meditation taught to help control the effects of stress and massage can be considered a very effective method of helping relaxation.

Aromatherapy massage is increasingly being used for clients who suffer from stress and stress-related symptoms.

The essential oils of plants that are used in aromatherapy are all volatile and have their own distinctive smells. The receptors for the sense of smell or olfaction are in the lining of the upper part of the nose. Olfactory nerves carry messages from these cells to a specific part of the brain where the impulses are interpreted as odour and give rise to the sensation of smell. The sensation of smell happens quickly. Adaptation to odours also occurs quickly so that we become accustomed to most smells (this accounts for failure to detect the smell of gas which accumulates slowly in a room). The sense of smell also 'tires' very quickly if it is exposed to too great a variety of smells one after the other.

The area of the brain where smell is registered is directly connected to a part of the base of the brain called the hypothalamus which is also connected to parts of the brain's limbic system, indeed it is often considered to be part of it. The limbic system includes areas of grey matter which control the emotional aspects of behaviour such as pain, pleasure, anger, rage and fear, also sorrow, sexual feelings, calmness and affection. The hypothalamus itself regulates other body activities through its control of the endocrine system and the autonomic nervous system. So in aromatherapy, for example, although essential oils affect the body by being absorbed into the blood stream, they can also affect the emotional responses by smell alone. This is particularly important since smell seems to trigger memories which may be happy or unhappy and affect the client's emotional responses.

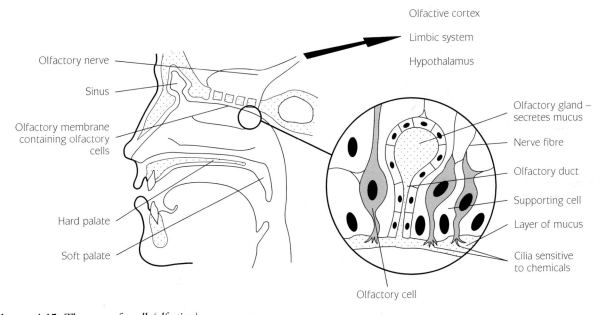

Figure 4.15 *The sense of smell (olfaction)*

ACTIVITY

Carry out a census among a group of friends to find out which perfumes they like and dislike. Ask them their reasons and discuss any memories they evoke or emotional responses.

The respiratory system

The respiratory system consists of the lungs and the tubes used for breathing.

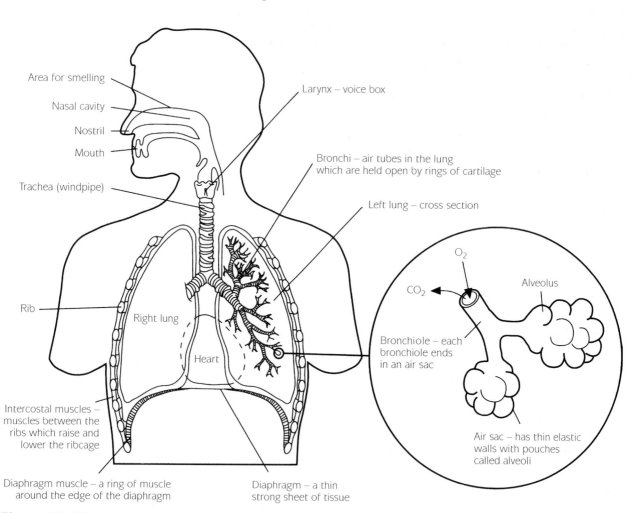

Area for smelling

Nasal cavity

Nostril

Mouth

Trachea (windpipe)

Larynx – voice box

Bronchi – air tubes in the lung which are held open by rings of cartilage

Left lung – cross section

O_2

CO_2

Alveolus

Bronchiole – each bronchiole ends in an air sac

Rib

Right lung

Heart

Air sac – has thin elastic walls with pouches called alveoli

Intercostal muscles – muscles between the ribs which raise and lower the ribcage

Diaphragm muscle – a ring of muscle around the edge of the diaphragm

Diaphragm – a thin strong sheet of tissue

Figure 4.16 *The respiratory system*

Air can be taken in either by the mouth or the nose, however the functions of the nose are particularly important in breathing. The nose:

- warms the air as it enters the body
- moistens the air

- traps dust and dirt
- smells odours.

Air passes along the windpipe (trachea) and bronchi to the two lungs which occupy the major volume of the chest cavity with the heart between them. The lungs are divided into lobes. The trachea divides into two bronchi, one to each lung, and the bronchi in turn divide into smaller and smaller tubes until the smallest, called bronchioles, end in air sacs called alveoli. The alveoli are bathed in blood and it is here that the exchange of gases between air and the blood takes place, supplying the body with oxygen and removing carbon dioxide.

A normal rate of breathing in an adult is between 14 and 18 times a minute. This increases with exercise or during some illnesses.

Asthma

Asthma is a reaction, often allergic, characterised by attacks of wheezing and difficult breathing. As dust or other airborne substances may trigger an attack, care must be taken with asthmatic clients not to expose them to substances which are allergens. It is sometimes necessary to position a client to help breathing and an asthmatic will nearly always be more comfortable sitting up than lying down.

Effects of massage on the respiratory system

- Vibratory or pounding movements over the chest wall may help to loosen secretions and to make the client cough.
- Some essential oils have specific effects on the respiratory system especially when inhaled.

Contraindications

to massage related to the respiratory system

- Any acute respiratory infections, for example colds, flu, or bronchitis.

Key Terms

You need to know what these words mean. Go back through the chapter or check in the glossary to find out.

- Allergens
- Alveoli
- Bronchioles

The digestive system

The digestive system consists of the alimentary canal, a long tube through which food passes, extending from the mouth to the anus and digestive glands which secrete digestive juices into the alimentary canal.

The digestive glands are as follows:

- salivary glands in the mouth
- gastric glands in the stomach

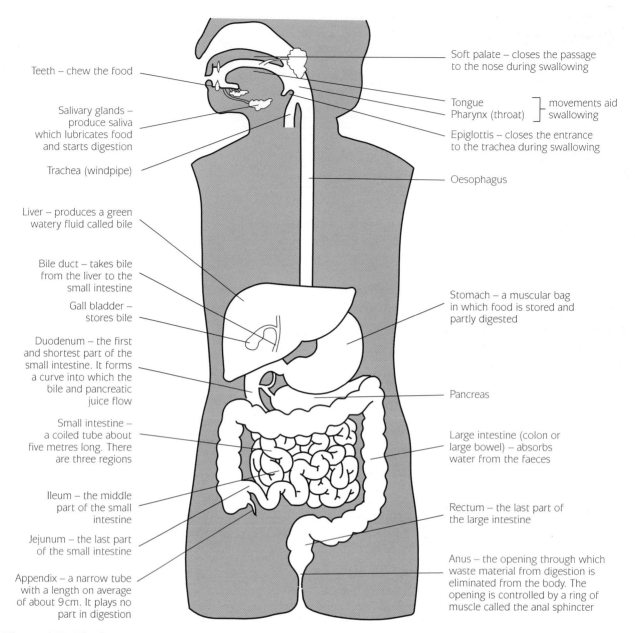

Teeth – chew the food

Salivary glands – produce saliva which lubricates food and starts digestion

Trachea (windpipe)

Liver – produces a green watery fluid called bile

Bile duct – takes bile from the liver to the small intestine

Gall bladder – stores bile

Duodenum – the first and shortest part of the small intestine. It forms a curve into which the bile and pancreatic juice flow

Small intestine – a coiled tube about five metres long. There are three regions

Ileum – the middle part of the small intestine

Jejunum – the last part of the small intestine

Appendix – a narrow tube with a length on average of about 9 cm. It plays no part in digestion

Soft palate – closes the passage to the nose during swallowing

Tongue
Pharynx (throat) } movements aid swallowing

Epiglottis – closes the entrance to the trachea during swallowing

Oesophagus

Stomach – a muscular bag in which food is stored and partly digested

Pancreas

Large intestine (colon or large bowel) – absorbs water from the faeces

Rectum – the last part of the large intestine

Anus – the opening through which waste material from digestion is eliminated from the body. The opening is controlled by a ring of muscle called the anal sphincter

Figure 4.17 *The digestive system*

- liver
- pancreas
- intestinal glands in the small intestine.

In the oesophagus, before the food reaches the stomach, and in the intestines after it has left the stomach, food is pushed along by rhythmic contractions called peristalsis. During an abdominal massage movements are performed over the lower part of the stomach and over the large and small intestine. It is important to know the position of these parts of the system as they are not protected by the skeleton and will be vulnerable to pressure being put on them.

Effects of massage on the digestive system

- Gentle movements over the large intestine in a clockwise direction may stimulate peristalsis and prevent constipation.

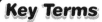
The renal system

The renal or urinary system consists of two kidneys, the tubes called ureters passing to the bladder, the bladder and the tube through which urine is expelled, the urethra.

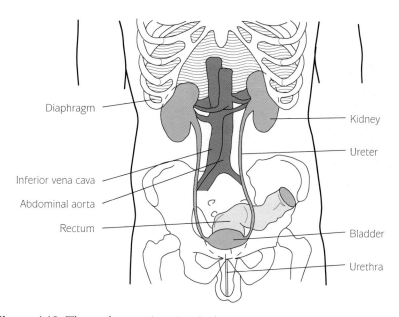

Figure 4.18 *The renal system (anterior view)*

Blood passes through the kidneys which remove unwanted substances from the blood and pass them in the form of urine to the bladder. When the pressure of urine in the bladder reaches a certain level it triggers a reflex to relax one of the muscles controlling the outlet. Another muscle is under voluntary control and can override the reflex to prevent urine being released until a convenient time.

The kidneys are delicate organs which are protected by the ribs, muscles of the back and a layer of fat surrounding them. However pressure over them can be very uncomfortable and massage movements such as beating and pounding must not be used in the area.

The bladder is situated behind the pubic bone and when empty looks like a deflated balloon. As urine volume increases it becomes pear shaped and rises up into the abdominal cavity. During massage any pressure over a full bladder will be intensely uncomfortable, therefore always suggest that a client empties the bladder before a body massage.

Effects of massage on the renal system

♦ Stimulation of the lymphatic system may increase the amount of urine passing to the bladder.

Contraindications

to massage related to the renal system

♦ Over the abdomen in someone who has had a kidney transplant.

Key Terms

You need to know what these words mean. Go back through the chapter or check in the glossary to find out.

♦ Reflex
♦ Renal
♦ Urinary

The endocrine system

The endocrine system is a control system of the body which works with the nervous system to maintain homeostasis. Homeostasis describes the state in which the body's internal environment stays constant. Whereas the nervous system controls the body by electrical impulses sent along nerves, the endocrine system works by releasing chemical messengers called hormones, into the blood stream.

The amount of hormone released by an endocrine gland is determined by the need for the hormone at any given time. The body is normally regulated so that there is no over or under production of hormones. There are times when the regulating mechanism does not operate properly and hormonal levels are too high or too low; when this happens endocrine disorders result. Some endocrine disorders which may be met by therapists are outlined below.

1 Hypothyroidism – too little output from the thyroid gland causes the body to retain water so that the face and body often look puffy, the skin looks thick and coarse and the hair is thin, dull and lifeless. Other symptoms may be lethargy and a tendency to gain weight. It is much more common in women than men. Women may fail to seek medical help because they assume that these symptoms indicate the onset of the menopause.
2 Hyperthyroidism – too much output from the thyroid gland causes weight loss, anxiety, tremor in the hands, increased sweating and a fast pulse.

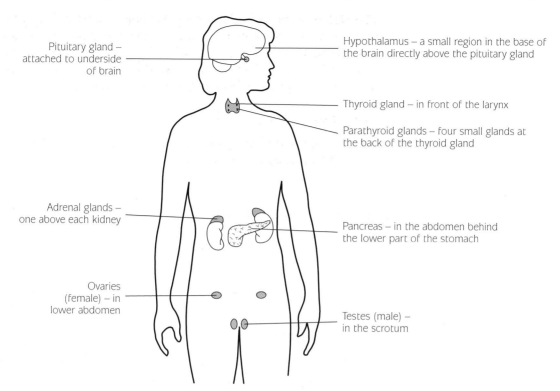

Figure 4.19 *The position of endocrine glands*

Endocrine gland	Hormone(s)	Action of hormone(s)
Pituitary gland	Growth hormone	Stimulates growth of bone and muscle
	Prolactin	Stimulates the breasts to produce milk in the female at the time of giving birth and afterwards maintains the milk supply
	Oxytocin	Stimulates the uterus in the female to contract at the end of pregnancy
The pituitary gland also produces hormones that control the function of all other endocrine glands		
Hypothalamus	Various	Control the pituitary gland
Thyroid gland	Thyroid hormones	Control metabolic rate
Parathyroid gland	Parathyroid hormone	Regulates the amount of calcium in the blood
Adrenal glands	Adrenaline (epinephrine)	Prepares the body for physical action
	Corticosteroids	Help to maintain homeostasis
Pancreas	Insulin	Reduces the level of glucose (sugar) in the blood
	Glucagon	Raises the level of glucose in the blood
Testes	Androgens (male sex hormones)	Control the development and function of the male sex organs and control development of secondary sexual characteristics
Ovaries	Oestrogens (female sex hormones)	Control the development and function of the female sex organs and control development of secondary sexual characteristics
	Progesterone	Prepares for and maintains pregnancy

Table 4.3 *Endocrine glands and the hormones they produce*

3   Diabetes – too little output of insulin from the pancreas results in glucose building up in the blood. There are different types of diabetes which affect 1–2 % of the population. People with

diabetes may have related conditions such as high blood pressure, other circulatory troubles, altered sensation in the limbs, eyesight problems and poor healing of the skin, especially in the feet.

ACTIVITY

Carry out some research to find out about other disorders of the endocrine system, especially those which might alter a person's appearance in some way.

Effects of massage on the endocrine system

General massage, by combating stress, can support the endocrine system in maintaining homeostasis. Some essential oils used in aromatherapy have an effect on the system either on the glands themselves or through the action of phytohormones (plant hormones) on the corresponding human hormones.

Contraindications

to massage related to the endocrine system

- ◆ Care must be taken when using massage on areas of the body which are particularly affected by diabetes.
- ◆ Some essential oils are contraindicated due to their hormonal actions particularly during pregnancy.

Stress

Massage and aromatherapy are often recommended for stress-related conditions. Therefore it is important to have some idea of the nature of stress.

Stress is any stimulus which creates a disturbance in the body that upsets homeostasis. Stress may be caused by:

- ◆ heat or cold
- ◆ noise
- ◆ worry about work or relationships
- ◆ pain or illness.

Most stresses are mild and routine. The body has many regulating devices which combat routine stress and 'balance' the body again. Stress only becomes harmful when it is continuous, difficult to cope with and when it disrupts normal life. Whether stress becomes harmful depends on the person's ability to cope, the amount of stress involved and the length of time the stress continues.

Too much stress can cause a state of anxiety or depression and produce feelings of fear and anger. These may, in turn cause physical symptoms in the body such as:

- ◆ headaches
- ◆ chest pain
- ◆ breathlessness
- ◆ skin rashes
- ◆ abdominal pain and indigestion

- irritability
- mood swings
- poor performance at work.

Stress over a long period of time may result in general adaptation syndrome, a condition where temporary changes become chronic and the general level of health declines.

Illnesses which may be associated with stress are:

- cardiovascular disease
- respiratory disease
- cancer
- depression
- stomach ulcers.

Stress can also depress the body's immune system.

The immune system

The essential function of the immune system is defence against infection. Immunity of the body to attack is obtained when the body produces antibodies in response to antigens

Antigens

Antigens are substances which stimulate the body to produce antibodies, for example bacteria, viruses, pollen and some foods. Antigens stimulate the activity of special lymphocytes called T-cells or B-cells. Antigens are found on the surfaces of foreign organisms, on the surface of red blood cells, on pollens, in poisons (toxins) and in foods.

Antibodies

Antibodies are made by white blood cells called lymphocytes and are found in the body tissues, blood and lymph nodes. They are proteins called immunoglobulins. Each different antigen stimulates the production of the particular type of antibody which will destroy that antigen.

Immunity can:

- be total when all the antigens are destroyed
- be partial when the antigens cause some reaction in the body
- fail when the antigens are not destroyed and infection or reaction follows.

There are different types of immunity.

1 Active immunity is when the body produces its own antibodies in response to either infection or a vaccine. Active immunity gives long-term immunity to specific diseases such as measles or poliomyelitis.
2 Passive immunity is when antibodies to specific diseases are injected. Passive immunity gives short-term protection against infections such as tetanus or hepatitis.
3 Inborn immunity occurs when the baby is in the uterus – antibodies from the mother cross into the baby's blood. The baby

is then protected against those diseases that the mother has had or been immunised against. This protection lasts for a few months after birth, when the baby is able to develop its own antibodies.

Autoimmune disease

Under normal circumstances, the body's immune system recognises its own tissues and chemicals but, if this recognition fails, the body produces antibodies which destroy its own cells. Examples of autoimmune diseases are some thyroid diseases, rheumatoid arthritis, and colitis.

Allergy

Allergy is an overreaction of the body against a substance to which it has become sensitive. Someone who is too reactive to an antigen is said to be allergic or hypersensitive. Antigens that induce an allergic reaction are called allergens. Examples of allergens are certain foods such as nuts or fruit, cosmetics, pollens and microbes. The first stage of allergy is sensitisation when the allergen first enters the body. The second exposure will cause cell damage.

Injured cells release histamine which causes tissue damage especially to smooth muscle cells (affecting breathing) and the permeability of blood vessels (causing oedema).

Anaphylactic shock is a severe allergic response that must be treated promptly with antihistamines or adrenaline.

If products are being used in a treatment, the client should always be asked about allergies. It is particularly important when using nut oils such as almond or peanut oil for massage as nut allergy is a growing problem.

People who have had an organ transplant, such as a kidney or heart transplant, have their immune system depressed by drugs to prevent the body's immune system from rejecting and destroying the new organ. Such people will have less resistance to infection.

Effects of massage on the immune system

Because of the calming effects of massage and its benefits in the treatment of stress, massage and aromatherapy are now thought to help to boost a depressed immune system. They are two of the complementary therapies being extensively used in diseases such as AIDS where the immune system is failing to cope with infection.

ACTIVITY

Find out which other complementary therapies are said to help stress-related conditions and look them up to see how their effect on stress-related problems is explained.

Key Terms

You need to know what these words mean. Go back through the chapter or check in the glossary to find out.

- Antibodies
- Antigens
- Autoimmune disease
- B-cells
- Endocrine
- Homeostasis
- Metabolic rate
- Phytohormones
- T-cells

After working through this chapter you will be able to:

- demonstrate suitable hand exercises for improving flexibility and strength
- demonstrate correct standing posture
- explain the importance of continuity, rhythm and depth
- obtain and react to client feedback
- describe and demonstrate the five major categories of massage
- describe the uses, points of care and contraindications specific to each category.

Massage is often called soft tissue manipulation. Soft tissue is a general term to cover all the superficial tissues other than bone, i.e. skin, fat, muscle and other connective tissue such as ligaments and tendons that may be affected by massage. While a knowledge of the structures of the body is important to develop and adapt massage, an in-depth knowledge is not absolutely essential when starting to learn. Ideally, the practical skills of massage and the theoretical knowledge of the structures and functions of the body should be studied together.

The hands are very sensitive and dextrous parts of the body so that while they are performing massage strokes they will also be receiving information about the body being worked on – information such as the temperature of the body, texture of the skin, firmness of the muscles, the relative thinness or fatness of the body and of course whether the hands are working over bony or soft tissue.

The sensitivity of the hands must be used to assess the state of the tissues and to learn about the client. It is a very direct form of feedback. If you cause pain or discomfort you should feel the client react and similarly if your touch is too light, many people will respond by tensing the area. A question such as 'Is that too deep?' will show that you are concentrating, thinking about the massage and are willing to adapt it to the individual client. This is a very important part of the caring process which enhances the client–therapist relationship.

Whenever possible, position yourself so that you can see the client's face to observe any reactions. Eventually, the adaptation of massage to the individual should become intuitive and almost automatic but never uncaring.

REMEMBER
It is easy to let your mind wander when massaging. The moment this happens the massage will suffer. Always concentrate on what you are doing.

There are three particularly important constituents of a good massage which should always be kept in mind.

- Continuity.
- Rhythm.
- Depth.

Continuity

Interruptions in the massage routine should be kept to a minimum with the hands staying in contact as much as possible and the transition from one stroke to another made without a break. This achieves continuity.

Rhythm

The rhythm should be even and steady with no jerkiness that would disturb the routine. The rate may be slow for relaxation or faster for more stimulation. Some therapists find music a help to set a mood but care must be taken not to try to fit the movements to the music. (Care should also be taken to check that the choice of music does not irritate the client.)

Depth

The depth of massage should be appropriate to the needs and physical state of the client. Thus the depth of massage used for a young fit person would be different from that used on someone who was elderly and frail. However, it should be remembered that most people prefer a firm massage and that, in the initial treatment, the client's reactions and opinions should be sought and recorded for future reference. The depth of the massage is altered by using the weight of your body effectively, so the posture and stance of the therapist and the height of the couch are of vital importance in performing effective massage.

GOOD PRACTICE

Stance

The therapist must be able to carry out any of the massage movements along the whole length of the part of the body being treated without strain. This can be achieved by taking up an effective working position and maintaining good posture. The feet should always be apart to provide a good base and help balance while working. The line between the feet should be in the same direction as the direction of movement. This enables the whole body to be moved in the direction of movement with the weight being transferred from one foot to the other. In the main, the feet should be in either the walk-standing position with one foot in front of the other or in stride-standing with the feet level but apart. The back should always be straight to reduce strain and the shoulders relaxed. The knees may be bent to reduce height instead of bending the back. Try to keep the arms out away from the body to help attain a relaxed movement.

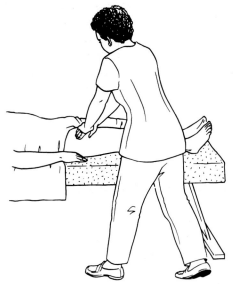

Figure 5.1 *Walk-standing: correct*

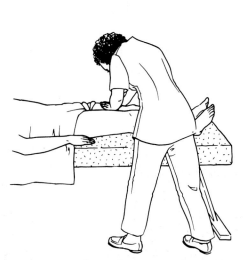

Figure 5.2 *Walk-standing: incorrect*

Hands

Hands must be relaxed and warm. Tension in the hands is soon detected by the client and can be very uncomfortable. The hands will be fully in contact with the body for the majority of the massage and need to be strong and flexible as well as being sensitive enough to assess the state of the tissues being worked on. The more massage is practised, the stronger and more flexible the hands become.

There are many simple exercises which could be carried out daily to help to mobilise and strengthen the hands and wrists. One such sequence of simple hand exercises is described below.

1   Hold the hands at chest level and shake them loosely and vigorously for a count of ten.
2   Touch the fingertips of one hand to the fingertips of the other and press so that the fingers and thumbs are widespread and pushed back. Bounce the fingers together to increase the range of movement in the fingers.
3   Place the palms of the hands together and lift the elbows so that the wrists are bent at right angles and press one hand against the other alternately back and forth to mobilise the wrists.
4   Lightly clench the hands at chest level and rotate the hands ten times in one direction then ten times in the other direction.
5   Clench and unclench the hands very quickly about ten times and then repeat the fist shaking exercise.

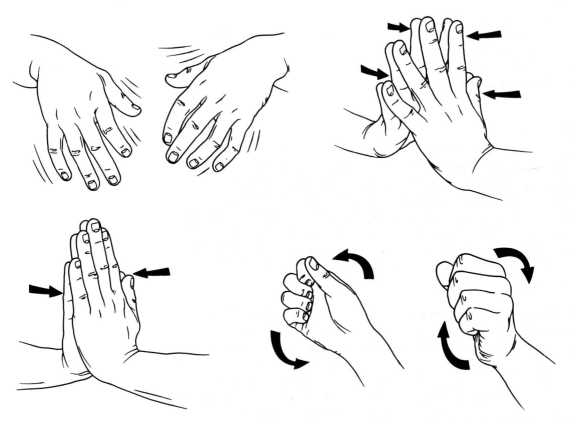

Figure 5.3 *Hand exercises*

Lubricant

Most therapists use some form of lubricant on the hands to prevent the hands dragging on the skin. Whatever lubricant is chosen, there should never be more than the minimum used: just enough to prevent dragging, but not enough to make the hands slip and slide with loss of control. More lubricant can be added during the massage if needed, but having to remove excess is disruptive. The choice of lubricant is between a cream, an oil or talcum powder and is discussed in chapter 2, 'The working environment'.

If you need to add oil during the massage, dribble a little on to the back of the hand which is on the body then pick the oil up by passing the other hand over it.

GOOD PRACTICE

Before you start a massage:

◆ make sure you have all the necessary equipment within reach
◆ check that everything is clean and hygienic
◆ warm and exercise your hands if necessary
◆ wash your hands.

The massage movements in this chapter are described in the traditional way in the following groups.

1 Effleurage and stroking.
2 Petrissage – to include kneading, picking up, wringing and rolling.
3 Tapotement (also called percussion).
4 Vibrations and shaking.
5 Friction and frictions.

Effleurage and stroking

The word 'effleurage' means 'to stroke', but the two terms have come to have slightly different meanings in massage today. In both movements, the hands move over the skin in the same manner. However, they differ in direction of movement. In effleurage, the movement is in the direction of the lymphatic and venous flow and so will affect the flow of blood and lymph in the vessels. Stroking is used to describe similar movements but direction is not important and rather than affecting the flow of blood and lymph it is mainly used for its sensory effects.

The rhythmic, flowing movements of effleurage and stroking are most important in a general massage. As they cover the whole area to be treated, these movements will be used to start and finish the massage, spread the chosen lubricant, link other strokes together and even to fill in a gap when you can't think what to do next! The speed and depth of the strokes in effleurage and stroking may be altered according to the effects desired. Slow deep strokes are relaxing while brisker, more superficial strokes tend to be stimulating.

Effleurage

Stance Walk-standing in the direction that the hands will move.

Hands One hand or two may be used depending on the size of the part to be treated. If one hand only is working, then the other can be used to support the part. Usually the whole surface of the palm and fingers is used but on very small areas the padded surface of the fingers and thumb may be used.

The hands and fingers should be relaxed and fit to the part so that they are in perfect contact with the skin. If any part of the hand is held stiffly then the effleurage strokes will feel hard and uncomfortable. To begin a stroke, the hands are placed on the end of the part of the body furthest away from the heart, the distal extremity, e.g. on the foot to begin effleurage to the leg or on the lower back at the start of effleurage to the back. The fingers should be pointing in the direction of movement, they are moved firmly upwards over the skin to cover the required area and then more lightly back down to the starting point.

Uses

- To start and finish massage to an area.
- To link between other strokes.
- To accustom the client to the therapist's touch.
- To spread the lubricant evenly.
- To warm the skin and produce an erythema.
- To induce relaxation and reduce muscle tone.
- To improve lymphatic and venous drainage.
- To remove dead skin cells, stimulate sweat and sebaceous glands and improve the suppleness of the skin.

> **REMEMBER**
> Physiological effects of massage are described in the previous chapter.

Stroking

Stance Walk-standing as for effleurage.

Hands Relaxed, moulded to the part and in full contact with the skin. The strokes may be in any direction over the skin, for example downwards as in returning from an effleurage movement on the back or leg, circular as in circling around the scapulae on the upper back or sideways as may be done at the waist. The depth and speed will vary according to the intensity of the effects required and occasionally one hand may be placed over the other to increase the depth; this is called reinforced stroking.

Uses

- To act as a link between other movements.
- To get the hands to a new position without breaking the continuity of the massage.
- To warm the area and produce an erythema.
- To aid relaxation and reduce muscle tone.
- To remove dead skin cells, stimulate sweat and sebaceous glands and improve the suppleness of the skin.

Points of care for effleurage and stroking

- Don't drag on the skin.
- Use more lubricant on hairy skin and whenever possible work with the natural lie of the hair. On very hairy skin omit effleurage completely.
- Lighten the pressure as the hands pass over bony or sensitive areas.

Contraindications

to effleurage and stroking

- Over any areas of skin showing signs of infection or skin conditions which may spread.
- Over any bruised area.
- Over obvious varicose veins which are painful or tender to the touch. Light strokes may be used over superficial veins that are not tender.
- Over an area where there has been a deep venous thrombosis or thrombophlebitis.

REMEMBER
Advice on medical referral is given in chapter 3, 'Consultation'.

ACTIVITY
Try the following practical exercises. (Note: the term 'client' is used throughout even though it is presumed that practice will take place on a colleague or other model.)

1 Effleurage to the back

With a client lying prone on a couch of suitable height, cover the legs and buttocks so that the length of the back is exposed. The client's arms may be loosely by the side or bent up with the hands beside the head.

Stance   By the side of the couch in walk-standing at the level of the client's hips so that you can reach the whole length of the back from the base of the spine to the neck. Your feet should be pointing towards the head of the couch.

Hands   Relaxed and warm with a little of the oil or lubricant spread on them. Place both hands on the lower back with fingers pointing up the back with the whole of the hands in contact. Now move both hands up the back, one on each side of the spine to the top of the back where the fingers will curl over the top of the shoulders. In order to reach the shoulders and keep the depth of the stroke even, you must move your body weight from the back foot to the front foot bending the front knee slightly.

Keeping contact, bring the hands back down to the base of the spine. The downward stroke should be lighter and more superficial than the upward stroke and be a little further out to the side. Repeat this movement a number of times until a rhythm is built up. Increase the depth on the upward effleurage movement but keep the speed steady and even. Move your weight from the back foot to the front foot in the upward movement, and use your body weight to apply pressure.

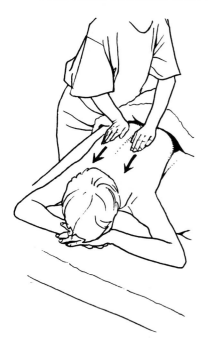
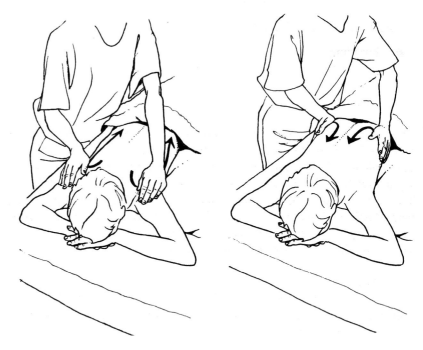

Figure 5.4 *Effleurage to the back*

2 Reinforced stroking

The client should be lying prone with the back exposed.

Stance Walk-standing at waist level facing the head of the couch.

Hands Make sure there is enough lubricant on the hands and place them between the scapulae with one hand over the other. Move both hands upwards between the bones, around one scapula and then the other in a figure-of-eight pattern. The pressure should be deeper on the upward movement and there should be no pressure at all as the hands cross the bony points of the spine.

REMEMBER
Keep the speed steady and even. Transfer body weight and maintain good posture.

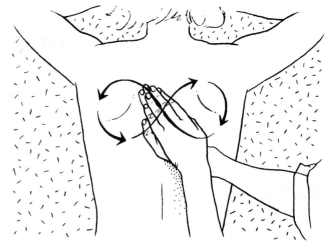

Figure 5.5 *Reinforced stroking to the back*

Petrissage

Petrissage movements are those in which soft tissues are compressed against underlying bone or squeezed in some way. The term 'kneading' is sometimes used to describe all petrissage movements but more correctly should only be used to describe compression against underlying bone.

Petrissage movements include:

- kneading
- picking up
- wringing
- rolling.

These squeezing, compressing movements have a pumping effect on the blood and lymphatic vessels in the soft tissues and stimulate the drainage of lymph and blood. Many of the petrissage movements will also put a slight stretch on the tissue, helping to maintain elasticity and mobility. This is particularly relevant for the superficial muscles where the massage may stretch the muscle fibres along their length as in wringing or across their width as in rolling. The movements will cause dilation of superficial blood vessels causing an erythema.

Kneading

Kneading is a circular movement where the hand moves the skin on the deeper tissues. The hands do not move over the skin except to move to the next part to be treated.

Stance Walk-standing in the direction of the main movement.

Hands Depending on the size of the area being treated, kneading can be performed with both hands at a time, or with one hand, or with a smaller part of the hand such as the palm or the thumbs. The pressure is varied, with greater pressure being applied on the upward part of the circle The pressure is increased by use of body weight. Both hands may be used together or alternately, or a single hand may be used with the other supporting the part. Where the tissues are dense and thick, one hand may be placed over the other to give extra force and depth to the movement, often called reinforced kneading.

Uses

- To stimulate lymphatic drainage in the muscles and other tissues.
- To stimulate the supply of arterial blood in the muscles and other tissues.
- To produce dilation of the superficial blood vessels (vaso-dilation) and erythema.
- To mobilise subcutaneous tissue.

Contraindications

to kneading

- Over bruised or tender areas.

1 Single-handed kneading to the thigh

The client should be lying supine with the leg nearest you uncovered.

Stance Walk-standing facing the head of the couch at knee level.

Hands A minimum amount of oil should be used as the hands must not slide on the skin. Place one hand on the inner surface of the knee for support. The other hand is placed on the outer surface of the upper thigh with the arm and elbow held well away from the side – this is the working hand. The outer, working hand is moved in a circular fashion on the outer thigh moving the skin over the deeper tissues. The circle should be made three or four times, then the hand should slide down the thigh a little and the circles repeated until the hand reaches to just above the knee. The movement can be repeated by sliding the hand up the outer thigh to the starting point. The outer hand then becomes the supporting hand while the inner hand repeats the movement down the inner thigh to the knee. Pressure will be lighter on the inside of the leg as the tissue is more sensitive.

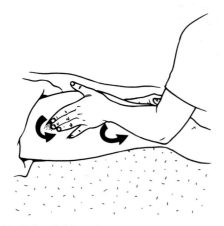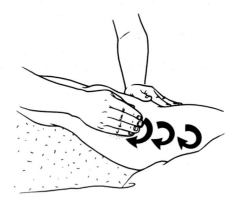

Figure 5.6 *Single-handed kneading*

2 Double-handed kneading

Stance As for single-handed kneading.

Hands One on the inside and one on the outside of the upper thigh – now both are working hands. The elbows should be bent and away from the sides so that the thigh is squeezed between both hands. The hands are moved alternately in a circular fashion, maintaining the squeezing effect and only moving over the skin to progress gradually down the leg to the knee. When the knee is reached, both the hands slide up the thigh to the starting position and the movement is repeated. This is quite hard work and needs practice to be able to do it without strain.

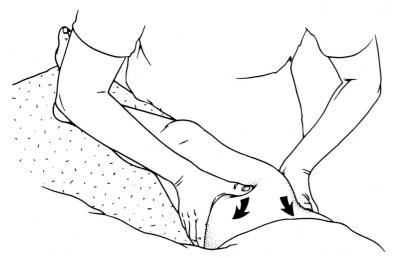

Figure 5.7 *Double-handed kneading*

> **REMEMBER**
> Don't hold your breath while working. This creates tension, which will affect the massage.

Picking up

Picking up is a petrissage movement where the soft tissue is picked up, lifted away from the deeper tissue or bone, squeezed and released.

Stance   Walk-standing in the direction of movement.

Hands   One hand or two may be used, but it is easier to start with one hand, using the other to support the part. In single-handed picking up, the part of the hand used is the V between the thumb and fingers. The tissues being worked on are lifted, squeezed and released. Be careful not to dig in with the fingers and thumb and keep the whole of the V as well as the palm in contact to avoid pinching. At the start of the movement, apply compression through the hand, then grasp the tissue and lift it away from the bone before releasing it and moving on.

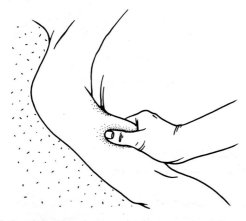

Figure 5.8 *Single-handed picking up*

Double-handed picking up is used on large muscular areas such as the front of the thigh where both hands are needed to span the muscle. The hands are arranged so that the thumb of one hand lies alongside the index finger of the other, forming a much wider V-shape with which to grasp the muscle. The action is the same – press, squeeze, lift, release and move on. The whole of the palms of the hands should be in contact.

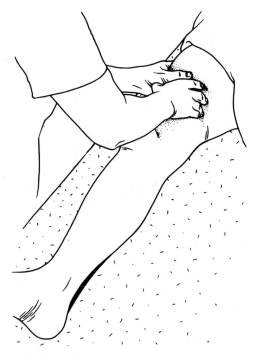

Figure 5.9 *Double-handed picking up*

Uses

◆ To stimulate venous and lymphatic flow.
◆ To stimulate arterial flow.
◆ To loosen tight subcutaneous tissue.

SAFE PRACTICE

Points of care
◆ Keep your palms in contact.
◆ Don't dig your fingers in.
◆ Keep your shoulders relaxed.

Contraindications
to picking up

◆ Over bruised or tender tissue.

ACTIVITY
Try the two following practical exercises for single- and double-handed picking up.

---

1 Single-handed picking up

On your own forearm, grasp the muscles on the thumb side of your forearm just below elbow level with the palm of the other hand so that the muscles fit into the V between thumb and forefinger. Lift the muscles away from the bone, squeeze, release and slide the hand a little lower and repeat until you reach just above the wrist. Slide the hand back up and repeat.

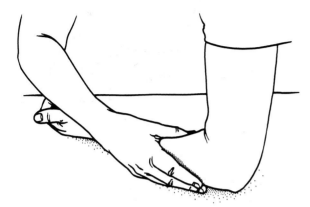

Figure 5.10 *Practising single-handed picking up*

2 Double-handed picking up on the front of the thigh

The client should be supine lying with one leg uncovered.

Stance   Walk-standing at knee level.

Hands   Place both hands on the front of the thigh with one hand overlapping the other as described. The V of the hands should be as wide as possible. With both hands, press down, grasp the large quadriceps muscle mass between the hands, lift away from the bone and gently release the pressure. Slide the hands a little lower down and repeat until you can feel that there is no more muscle mass just above the knee. To reach the top of the thigh again, the hands can slide up or can repeat the picking up with the hands moving upwards.

Wringing

This is a petrissage movement similar to picking up. The tissues are compressed and picked up from the bone as in picking up, but instead of then being released they are passed from hand to hand in a wringing movement.

Stance   Stride-standing or walk-standing facing across the area to be treated.

Hands   Wringing is always performed with both hands. They are placed on the part with the fingers on one side and the thumbs on the other. The arms must be held well out to the sides with the elbows half bent. Muscle and superficial tissue is compressed and scooped up between the fingers and thumb of each hand, then the fingers of one hand pull the tissue towards you while the thumb of the other hand pushes it away. The hands move along the length of the muscle wringing as they go. The smaller the

> **REMEMBER**
> Don't hunch your shoulders – it is very tiring.

muscle that is being worked on the more the fingers are used rather than the whole hand, for example across the shoulders where there is no room for the whole hand.

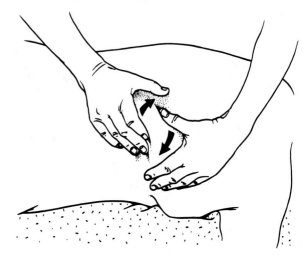

Figure 5.11 *Wringing on superficial tissue*

Uses

♦ To improve elasticity by stretching along the length of muscle.
♦ To soften hard subcutaneous fatty tissue.
♦ To improve local circulation.

Contraindications
to wringing

♦ Bruised or tender tissue.
♦ Areas of stretched skin.
♦ Areas of poor muscle tone, for example on an older client.

ACTIVITY
Try the following practical exercises for wringing.

1 Wringing to the muscles of the thigh
Stance Stride-standing facing across the client.

Hands Both on the upper inner thigh with fingers together and thumbs wide apart. Pick up the muscle with one hand then the other and start wringing by pulling with the fingers of one hand and at the same time pushing away with the thumb of the other hand. The movement is reversed so that the muscle is kept lifted away from the bone and is passed from hand to hand. Move the hands down the inner thigh, up the front of the thigh and down the outer surface wringing all the time. To reach the outer surface you must bend your knees to get your height down to the necessary level.

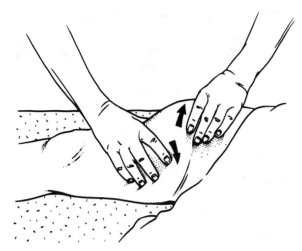

Figure 5.12 *Wringing to the muscles of the thigh*

2 Wringing to the shoulders
The client must be lying prone with the upper back exposed

Stance Walk-standing facing the head of the couch.

Hands Cupped over the shoulder furthest away from you. Pick up the muscle at the top of the shoulder between the fingers and thumb of both hands and wring the muscle by pulling with the fingers of one hand and pushing with the thumb of the other. Move the hands across the shoulder towards the neck. When the neck is reached, keep one hand in contact while the other moves across to the other shoulder. Follow with the other hand and continue wringing across to the point of the near shoulder. This can be repeated back and forth across the tops of the shoulders.

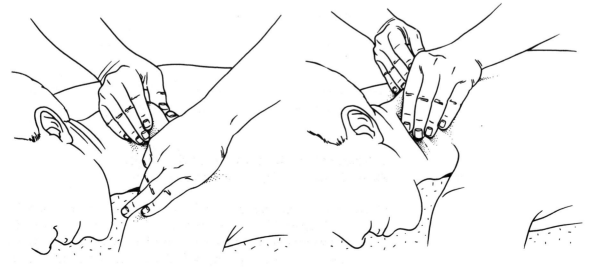

Figure 5.13 *Wringing to the shoulders*

Rolling

The most common type of rolling is skin rolling where the skin and subcutaneous tissue is rolled between fingers and thumb. Muscle rolling can be performed as a deeper form of the movement across muscle fibres.

Skin rolling

Stance   Facing across the part to be treated with the feet in walk- or stride-standing.

Hands   Placed flat on the part with the thumbs spread wide and their tips touching.

The fingers pull the tissue up into a roll against the thumbs which then push the roll of skin back towards the fingers. Keep a steady rhythm as the hands move up and down the area to be treated. This movement is easy when performed on the opposite side of the body from the therapist, i.e. pushing the roll of skin away with the thumbs, but is more difficult when being performed on the side nearest the therapist. Here the therapist can either twist the upper body and arms so that the movement can be carried out as before or reverse the hand movement so that the fingers push a roll of skin towards the thumbs.

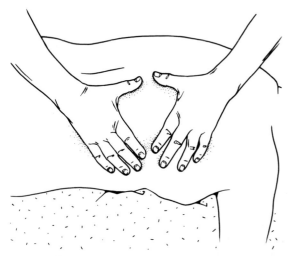

Figure 5.14 *Skin rolling: hand position*

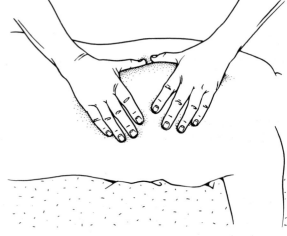

Figure 5.15 *Skin rolling: pulling the tissue into a roll with the fingers*

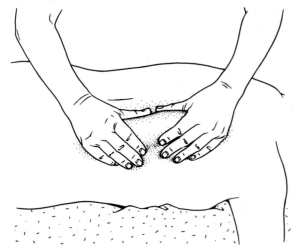

Figure 5.16 *Skin rolling: squeeze and lift*

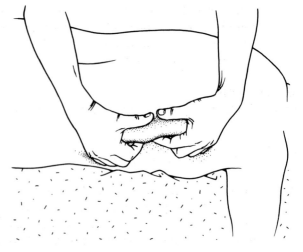

Figure 5.17 *Skin rolling: pushing the roll back with the thumbs*

Uses

- To stimulate the circulation of the skin.
- To soften hard subcutaneous tissue such as fat.
- To induce relaxation by the rhythmic nature of the strokes.
- To improve elasticity of the skin.
- To soften an area around old scar tissue.

Contraindications

to skin rolling

- Over an area of stretched or loose skin.
- Over bruised or tender skin.

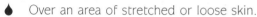

ACTIVITY

Try the following practical exercise for skin rolling.

Skin rolling to the back

The client should be lying prone with the back exposed.

Stance Walk-standing facing across client just above waist level.

Hands Placed on the side of the back away from you at the client's waist. The fingers should be straight with the thumbs as far away from the forefinger as possible. The tips of the thumbs should be touching and those of the forefingers almost touching. With the flat of the hand in contact with the skin, pull the fingers towards you so that the skin moves with them, press down with your thumbs and push the resulting roll of skin towards the fingers with the long surface of the thumbs. Repeat the movement in a smooth rhythm up and down the side of the body.

> **REMEMBER**
> Keep your back straight – bend your knees to reduce your height.

Muscle rolling

This is similar to skin rolling but is deeper and works across the fibres of a muscle.

Stance The same as for skin rolling.

Hands Placed in a similar position as for skin rolling but over a suitable muscle. The fingers and thumbs are pressed down so that the muscle bulges between them. The thumbs are rolled towards the fingers across the muscle fibres or slightly along them, whichever is most comfortable for the client.

♦ To relieve tension and adhesions in the muscle.
♦ To improve circulation in the muscle.

Points of care and contraindications are the same as for skin rolling.

> **ACTIVITY**
> Try the following exercise for muscle rolling.

Muscle rolling to the erector spinae
The client should lying prone face with the back uncovered.

Stance Walk-standing facing across the client at chest level.

Hands Place the hands flat on the far side of the back with the thumbs lying in the groove between the spine and the long muscle of the back [erector spinae]. With the fingers, feel for the far boundary of the muscle. Press firmly with the thumbs and fingers so that the muscle bulges between them and push across the muscle with the thumbs. Repeat down the length of the muscle to the base of the spine. To perform this movement on the side nearest you, you have to move the fingers towards the thumbs or work from the opposite side of the body.

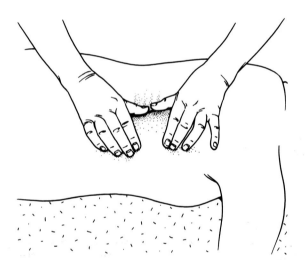
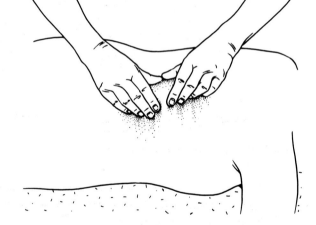

Figure 5.18 *Muscle rolling*

Tapotement/percussion

The terms 'tapotement' and 'percussion' are interchangeable and, as the names suggest, describe a group of movements where the parts are struck repeatedly with soft blows of the hands. Both hands are usually used and they strike the part alternately. The movements must be light and bouncy not heavy and solid. Practice is needed to achieve this and to acquire an easy, non-tiring rhythm. The wrists must be loose and the arms relaxed. There is always a tendency to hunch your shoulders and hold your breath when trying these movements.

All the movements are stimulating and are usually omitted from a relaxing style massage.

Tapotement/percussion movements are:

- ♦ Hacking.
- ♦ Pounding.
- ♦ Clapping.
- ♦ Beating.

The easiest way to practise all percussion movements is on a pillow or cushion placed on the treatment couch. This allows you to adjust the depth and rhythm until you feel confident enough to try them on a client.

Hacking

Stance   Walk-standing facing across the part to be treated.

Hands   Hacking is performed with a small part of the ulnar (little finger) side of the hands and the back of the little, ring and middle fingers. The elbows are bent and held well away from the body and the wrists are bent back as far as possible. The fingers should be loose, slightly apart and a little bent.

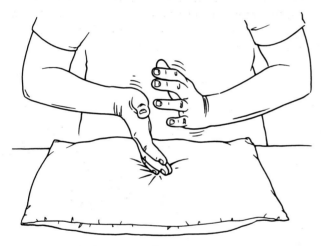

Figure 5.19 *Practising hacking on a pillow*

The movement is produced by rapidly striking the part with alternate hands Only the forearms and wrists move, not the shoulders or elbows. It should be rapid and light, making a tapping sound. On more muscular areas it can be a little slower and deeper.

Uses

- ♦ To stimulate superficial circulation and produce an erythema.
- ♦ To stimulate superficial muscle by producing a reflex contraction.

SAFE PRACTICE

Points of care for hacking
- ♦ Never use the whole side of the hand; it will be painful.
- ♦ Always avoid bony areas or those with little subcutaneous tissue.

ACTIVITY

Try the following practical exercise for hacking.

Hacking

With a pillow on the couch.

Stance   Stride-standing facing the couch.

Hands   Rest the ulnar (little finger) side of the hands on the pillow with the palms facing each other, the hands relaxed and only a little way apart. Bend the elbows to a right angle and take them away from your body. The wrists now should be fully extended. Keeping the elbows still, strike the pillow with alternate hands. Only the sides and backs of the little, ring and middle fingers and a small part of the side of the hand should strike the pillow. The striking should be so light as to almost flick the pillow rather than hit it.

When you have a steady rhythm, move the hands to cover the whole surface of the pillow and try to vary the speed and depth.

Pounding

This is a heavier percussion movement than hacking and should only be used over large, well covered areas such as the gluteal region.

Stance   The same as for hacking.

Hands   The elbows and arms are held in the same position as for hacking but the hands should be loosely clenched so that a soft fist is made. The movement made is similar to hacking, using alternate hands to strike the part with the side of the loose fist.

Uses

- To increase local circulation.
- To soften fatty tissue.

SAFE PRACTICE

Points of care for pounding

- Never clench fists tightly.
- Keep the wrists loose.

Pounding

Using a pillow, with loosely clenched fists perform the same movement as for hacking.

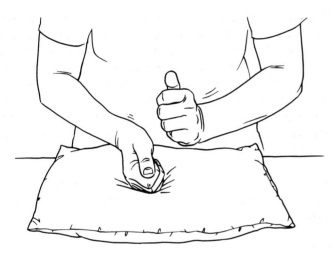

Figure 5.20 *Practising pounding on a pillow*

Clapping

Clapping is a percussion movement in which the area is struck with the hands cupped.

Stance Face across the part to be treated with the feet in walk- or stride-standing.

Hands Athough the palms of the hands are used to perform this movement, the hands should be cupped so that the centre of the palm does not touch the part. The fingers are held straight with the thumbs held close to the index fingers. The arms are held away from the sides of the body to allow for some movement at the elbows, although most of the movement takes place at the wrists. The hands strike the part alternately and should produce a dull, hollow sound, not a slapping noise.

Uses

- To stimulate skin circulation.
- To shake deeper tissues and stimulate circulation.

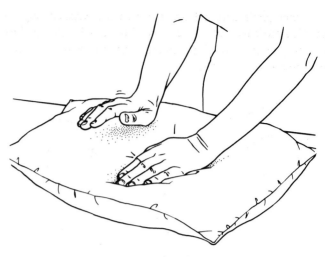

Figure 5.21 *Practising clapping on a pillow*

SAFE PRACTICE

Points of care for clapping
 Over sensitive skin, the movement may be performed over a towel or blanket.

Contraindications
to clapping

● Over bruised or tender skin.

ACTIVITY
Try the following exercise for clapping.

REMEMBER
If you lose the rhythm of the strokes, change to another stroke for a while then try again.

Clapping

Stance Walk- or stride-standing facing the pillow on the couch.

Hands Place both hands palm down on the pillow and draw up the centre of the hand until middle of the palm is off the pillow. Start to strike the pillow with alternate hands moving along the length of the pillow with the hands staying quite close to each other.

Beating

Beating is a percussion movement performed as in clapping but with the hands held in loose fists.

Stance Facing across the part to be treated with the feet in walk- or stride-standing.

Hands Held in loose fists but with the ends of the fingers held straight instead of tucked into the fist (this provides the flat surface to strike the part). The thumbs are kept close to the side of the fist and the wrists kept very loose.

The therapist's arms are lifted so that the wrists droop then the part is struck with alternate fists. This may be changed to clapping by just opening and cupping the hand. The arm movement remains the same.

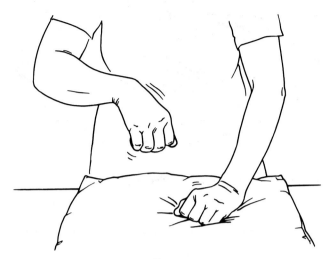

Figure 5.22 *Practising beating on a pillow*

Uses

◆ To soften hard fatty tissue.

Contraindications
to beating

◆ Over bruised or tender areas.
◆ Over weak muscles.

ACTIVITY
Try the following exercise for beating.

Beating
Repeat the exercise given for clapping but with the hand loosely clenched and the fingers straight.

Vibrations and shaking

These types of movements involve producing a tremor or shake in the tissues. However, the techniques they employ and their uses are very different.

Vibrations

In the vibrations movement, the effects are produced by the therapist vibrating the hands or fingers so that the vibrations are transmitted to the part being treated. The tremor may be produced by an up-and-down or side-to-side movement. It is difficult to do well and takes considerable practice.

Stance   Walk-standing facing across or along the part.

Hands   Only one hand works while the other supports the part. The arm is held outstretched and the hand placed firmly on the part. Either the whole hand with fingers and thumb close together or the tips of the fingers may be used. The hand and/or fingers are vibrated up and down to produce a fine tremor in the tissue or vibrated sideways to and fro the hand always keeping in contact with the skin.

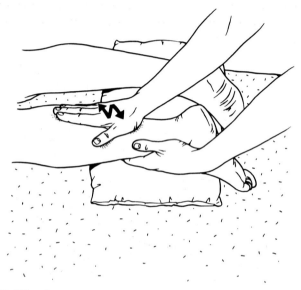

Figure 5.23 *Vibrations*

Uses

- Over the course of a nerve as a soothing mechanism.
- Over an area needing stimulation of lymphatic drainage.

SAFE PRACTICE

Points of care for vibrations
- Don't dig in with the fingertips.

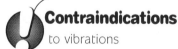 **Contraindications**
to vibrations
- Over very poorly covered areas.

ACTIVITY
Try the following exercise for vibrations.

Vibrations to the back of the thigh

The client should be lying prone with the back of one leg exposed.

Stance   Walk-standing facing the head of the couch at knee level.

Hands   Place the working hand flat, high up in the centre of the back of the thigh. The other hand rests on the side of the thigh to support it. Keeping the working arm outstretched, vibrate the hand up and down quite quickly and at the same time slide the hand down the centre of the back of the thigh to the level of the knee.

Shaking

This is a much less fine movement than vibrations. The muscle area being treated is grasped by the hand or fingers, usually towards the origin or insertion of the muscle, and then loosely shaken from side to side. In sports massage and sometimes shiatsu treatments, the whole limb may be shaken by grasping the hand or foot and shaking the whole arm or leg sideways or up and down.

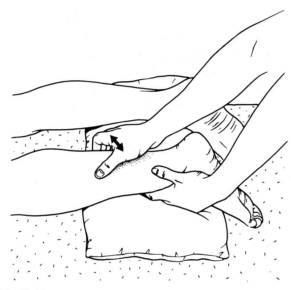

Figure 5.24 *Shaking*

Uses

◆   To relax the muscles.

> **REMEMBER**
> It helps the therapist to relax the shoulders occasionally while working. Do this by pushing them down to stretch the neck and then letting them spring back.

SAFE PRACTICE

Points of care for shaking
◆   Keep fingers as straight as possible to avoid digging in with the fingers.

Contraindications

to shaking

◆   Over thin or over-stretched muscles.

Friction and frictions

Although the names of the friction and frictions movements sound almost the same they are completely different and are described together here in order to stress the differences. Friction is the fast rubbing of the skin, often used to warm the skin, whilst frictions are small deep movements on localised areas which move superficial tissues on deep ones. Friction may be described as a fast stroking movement and frictions as deep petrissage.

Friction

Stance Walk- or stride-standing facing in the direction of general movement.

Hands The flat palmar surface of hands and fingers are used with the hands held stiffly so that the palm and fingers are firm. The hands are rubbed quickly over the skin in any direction.

Uses

- To stimulate the local blood supply.
- To warm the area being treated.

Contraindications
to friction

- Over very sensitive skin.
- Over very hairy skin.

ACTIVITY
Try the following exercise for friction.

Friction to the back

The client should be lying prone with the back uncovered.

Stance Walk-standing facing the head of the couch at waist level.

Hands Place flat on the back and hold stiff and firm, then, moving the hands briskly, rub the surface of the whole back in short random movements.

Frictions

Stance Walk- or stride-standing close to the couch to be able to exert enough force.

Hands The fingertips are used to apply frictions and the fingers must be held stiffly. The fingertips press firmly and move in small circles with no sliding over the skin. To move on lift the fingers, move to the next area, and continue. Small to-and-fro frictions are sometimes applied across particular muscle fibres. In each case superficial tissue is compressed and moved over the deeper tissues.

Uses

- To produce a localised erythema.
- To soften and stretch tight tissue such as scar tissue or adhesions in muscle.
- To ease the condition known as fibrositis which can be felt as hard bands of muscle fibres especially in the upper back.
- To stimulate the spinal nerves when used down the sides of the spine.
- In sports massage over ligaments.

Contraindications

to frictions

- Over painful areas.
- Over bony points.
- Over any area of inflammation.

ACTIVITY
Try the following exercise for frictions.

Frictions to the back
The client should be lying face down with the back uncovered.

Stance Walk-standing close to the couch at waist level.

Hands Place the middle finger of the working hand on the upper back just to the side of the spine and feel for the slight hollow where the fingertip fits naturally. Keep the finger straight, supporting it if necessary with the index finger and move the fingertip in small circles, moving the skin on the deeper tissue. Start quite lightly and gradually increase the depth. Work for five to ten circles before lifting the finger and moving down to the next hollow. The resting hand should be supporting the side of the back.

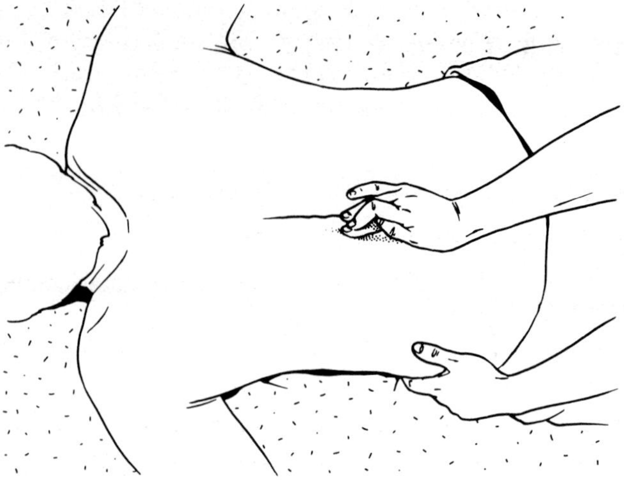

REMEMBER

The fingers receive information – take note of any reaction such as tensing the area to be treated.

Figure 5.25 *Frictions to the back*

Key Terms

You need to know what these words mean. Go back through the chapter or check in the glossary to find out.

- Distal
- Effleurage
- Friction
- Frictions
- Petrissage
- Prone
- Stroking
- Supine
- Tapotement
- Ulnar

THE MASSAGE ROUTINE

6

After working through this chapter you will be able to:
- prepare a client for a full body massage
- perform a full body massage using a suitable range of massage strokes
- determine and adapt the timing of massage for a whole body massage
- determine and adapt the timing of massage to particular areas
- obtain and appreciate the importance of client feedback.

In order to perform a body massage, the movements described in the previous chapter must be applied in some sort of order to the parts of the body to be treated. When starting to massage whole areas of the body rather than just practising a variety of strokes, it is important to have a few basic rules to follow. In the main, the first type of massage to be mastered should be a classic general purpose massage as this is the type of massage which contains most of the strokes needed. Once you are proficient at this it can then be adapted for any other purpose.

For example a relaxing body massage is one where the majority of strokes are of the effleurage and stroking type with some petrissage, while a more stimulating massage will contain percussion movements and more vigorous petrissage. The speed and depth of the strokes will also vary from slow and relaxing to faster and more invigorating, but, whatever the purpose of the massage, the strokes must always show continuity and rhythm and be at a depth suitable for the client being treated. The actual massage routine – that is the order of treating the parts of the body and the strokes used – is something that is altered to suit particular clients and to suit the preference of the therapist. Each expert massage therapist will have developed their own routines which are adapted and altered as part of a continual learning process. If you were to ask an expert to show you the massage movements that they used when they started, most would have difficulty in recalling them. However, they would have initially have learnt the strokes, or very similar ones, described in the previous chapter and will have developed, varied, adapted and linked them together to make up massage routines for any part of the body.

The massage routine described in this chapter is a general 'all purpose' one which is suitable to learn initially, remembering that it can be altered and adapted to suit yourself and your client. It is a routine that uses the majority of the previously described strokes and therefore would have to be adapted to be a completely relaxing massage by leaving out the percussion movements and reducing the more vigorous petrissage movements.

Before attempting a full body massage, the therapist should practise all the strokes on one particular part of the body until proficient before passing on to the next part. When you are proficient on each individual area then you can put it all together to perform a full body massage.

Whatever massage routine you will be performing, once it has started, that is once you have placed your hands on the client's body, then nothing should be allowed to disturb this continuity of the massage. This means, of course, that you must arrange your work so that you will not be disturbed by outside matters and that you have everything to hand so that you do not have to interrupt the massage to fetch anything. The preparation of the working area and the selection of suitable materials is described earlier, as is the consultation procedure. When everything is ready and the client is lying comfortably on the couch, then the massage can be started, remembering that only the part to be worked on should be uncovered as the rest of the body can quickly become chilled. Of course, in very hot and humid climates this would not apply and here a very light cover can be used.

Timing a massage treatment can be very difficult and it takes a long time for it to become automatic. To begin with, it is quite useful to time each individual part of the massage. If we assume that a full body massage will take an hour, not including the time taken for the client to prepare or to recover, then we can also suggest the time for each part within a routine. These times too, of course, will be altered and adapted to suit individual clients.

The following suggested routine is suitable to use to start with and can be adapted and altered to suit the client or your preference.

The following is a SUGGESTED OUTLINE and approximate times for a one-hour massage.

Client lies supine with head supported by a pillow.

1	Right leg	7 minutes
2	Left leg	7 minutes
3	Left arm	5 minutes
4	Chest	5 minutes
5	Right arm	5 minutes
6	Abdomen	5 minutes

Client turns over to lie prone, the pillow is removed.

7	Back of right leg including the buttock	5 minutes
8	Back of left leg including the buttock	5 minutes
9	Back and shoulders	15 minutes

This order of massage presumes that you are free to move around the couch as you wish. Occasionally you might find yourself trying to carry out massage with a couch pushed up against a wall and then everything has to change!

Movement by the therapist should be kept to a minimum and, wherever possible, contact with the client maintained. In general, the order of strokes to each area should be effleurage and stroking movements to start, followed by a variety of petrissage movements, then percussion to suitable parts and effleurage and stroking to complete before moving on to the next section of the massage.

To start the general massage the client should be lying on the couch with support under the head and covered by towels in such a way as to allow access to each area of the body to be treated with as little disturbance as possible. One method is to have one towel lengthways across the top of the body and another lengthways along the legs and lower trunk.

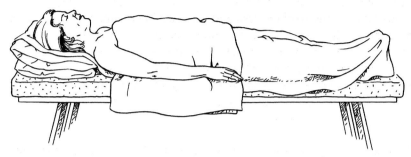

Figure 6.1 *Preparing the client for massage*

Numbers of repetitions of the strokes are not always given as this depends on the preference of the therapist and the specific needs of the client. To begin with, you can aim to repeat each movement three or four times so long as this fits in to the timing for the area.

Leg massage

The following are SUGGESTED MASSAGE MOVEMENTS for the right and left leg.

1. Effleurage to the sides and front of the whole of the leg.
2. Effleurage to the thigh.
3. Double-handed kneading to the thigh.
4. Single-handed kneading to the thigh.
5. Wringing to the thigh muscles.
6. Hacking to the thigh muscles.
7. Stroking around the knee.
8. Effleurage to the back of the calf with knee bent.
9. Effleurage to the lower leg.
10. Single-handed kneading to the anterior tibial muscles.
11. Effleurage to the foot.
12. Kneading to the sole of the foot.
13. Single-handed hacking to the sole of the foot.
14. Thumb stroking to the top of the foot.
15. Thumb stroking across the sole of the foot.
16. Kneading to the toes.
17. Repeat of effleurage to the front and sides of the whole leg.

ACTIVITY

Before starting the massage, remind yourself of the bony points to be avoided in the leg.

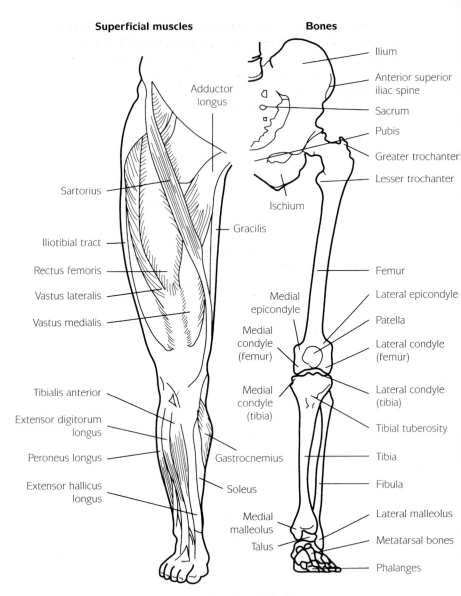

Superficial muscles

- Adductor longus
- Sartorius
- Gracilis
- Iliotibial tract
- Rectus femoris
- Vastus lateralis
- Vastus medialis
- Tibialis anterior
- Extensor digitorum longus
- Peroneus longus
- Extensor hallicus longus
- Gastrocnemius
- Soleus
- Medial malleolus

Bones

- Ilium
- Anterior superior iliac spine
- Sacrum
- Pubis
- Greater trochanter
- Lesser trochanter
- Ischium
- Femur
- Medial epicondyle
- Lateral epicondyle
- Patella
- Medial condyle (femur)
- Lateral condyle (femur)
- Medial condyle (tibia)
- Lateral condyle (tibia)
- Tibial tuberosity
- Tibia
- Fibula
- Lateral malleolus
- Metatarsal bones
- Phalanges
- Talus

Figure 6.2 *Muscles and bones of the front of the leg*

> **REMEMBER**
> Apply only enough oil to allow your hands to slide smoothly.

Fold the lower towel back to expose the whole of the right leg. Place some of the lubricant on the hands and apply it to the whole leg with sweeping effleurage-type strokes.

1 Effleurage to the sides and front of leg

Stance Walk-standing at the approximate level of the ankle making sure that you can reach to the top of the leg without straining.

Hands Place the hands on the foot, one hand under the sole and the other on the top so that the foot is held between the hands.

Slide the hands firmly up the foot so that the top hand comes to the outside and the lower hand to the inside of the ankle and continue with the effleurage stroke up the inside and outside of the leg to the top of the thigh, when the outside hand sweeps firmly over the top of the leg towards the groin and the inguinal lymph nodes. Return the hands to the starting position by reversing the stroke but with much less pressure. Repeat two or three times.

The next effleurage stroke starts in the same way with the hands cradling the foot and then sliding up the sides of the lower leg, but just above the level of the knee they are brought in to overlap each other on top of the thigh and sweep up to the groin area. Return the hands to the starting position with one on the inside and the other on the outside of the leg in the same way and repeat two or three times.

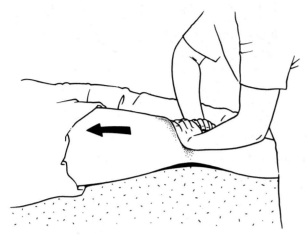

Figure 6.3 *Effleurage to the sides and front of the leg*

2 Effleurage to the thigh

Stance   Walk-standing at a little below knee level.

Hands   **a)** One inside and other outside the thigh above the knee.

Effleurage as before from knee to groin with the outer hand sweeping over the top of the thigh towards the inguinal nodes.

Hands   **b)** Overlapping each other above the knee sweeping up to the groin and returning to the knee level on the inside and outside of the thigh.

3 Double-handed kneading to the thigh

(This movement is described on pages 62–63, chapter 5.)

Stance   Walk-standing just below the level of the knee.

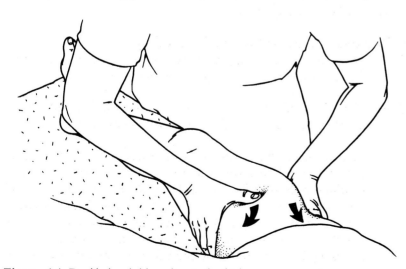

Figure 6.4 *Double-handed kneading to the thigh*

Hands Place one hand on the inside of the upper thigh and the other on the outside with the elbows bent and well away from the sides so that the thigh is squeezed between them. Move the hands alternately in circles away from you maintaining the squeezing effect and only moving over the skin to progress down the thigh to the knee. The hands can then slide back up the thigh to start again. Repeat two or three times.

4 Single-handed kneading to the thigh
(This movement is described on page 62, chapter 5.)

Stance Walk-standing just below the level of the knee.

Hands The working hand is placed on the outside of the upper thigh and the other hand on the inner thigh for support.

The working hand is moved in a circular fashion on the outer thigh, moving the skin over the deeper tissues. The circle should be made three or four times before sliding down a little to repeat the circling. When the level of the knee is reached, the hand slides up to the start. Repeat two or three times.

> **REMEMBER**
> Keep the whole hand in contact but do not to press too hard over the trochanter of the femur.

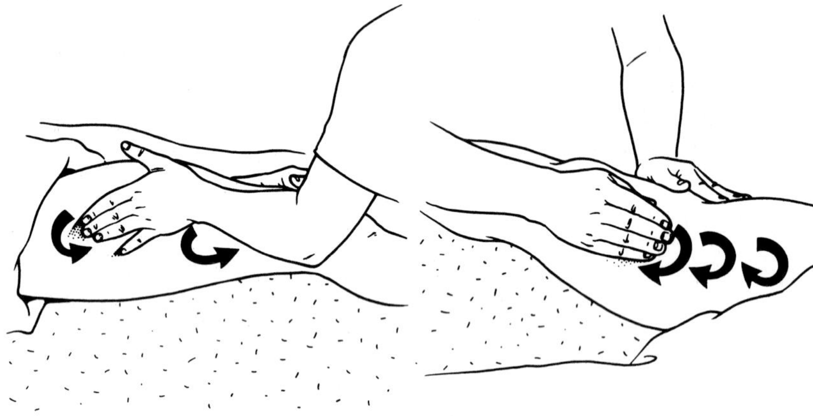

Figure 6.5 *Single-handed kneading to the thigh*

5 Wringing to the muscles of the thigh
(This movement is described on pages 66–67, chapter 5.)

Stance Walk- or stride-standing facing across the client.

Hands Placed on inner thigh facing each other with fingers together and thumbs apart.

Pick up the muscle on the inside of the thigh with one hand and then with the other and start the wringing movement by pulling with the fingers of one hand and pushing with the thumb of the other. The tissue is kept lifted from the bone as the hands wring and move up and down the thigh, first on the inside then on the top and then on the outside to cover the whole thigh.

> **REMEMBER**
> Bend your knees in order to reduce your height to work on the outside of the leg.

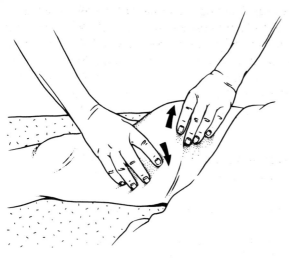

Figure 6.6 *Wringing to the muscles of the thigh*

6 Hacking to the thigh muscles

Stance   Stride-standing facing across the client.

Hands   Relaxed and with the palms facing each other a little way apart. The elbows should be bent and well away from the body.

Start hacking lightly down the front of the thigh and up again repeating so that the front and outer surface of the thigh are covered two or three times. The inner surface should be avoided as the tissue can be too sensitive for hacking.

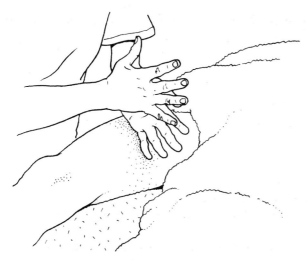

Figure 6.7 *Hacking to the thigh muscles*

Before moving on to the knee, effleurage over the thigh once or twice.

7 Stroking around the knee

Stance   Walk-standing below knee level.

Hands   Placed with the thumbs overlapping below the patella and the fingers resting at the sides of the knee.

The thumbs stroke up lightly over the patella and then sweep firmly around the edges of the patella and down towards the back of the knee to meet the fingers at the sides. Repeat two or three times.

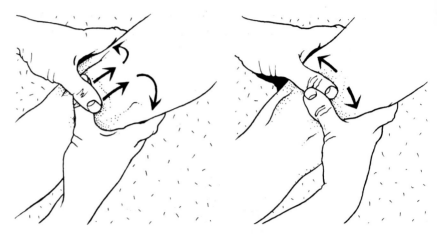

Figure 6.8 *Stroking around the knees*

8 Effleurage to the back of the calf
With one hand under the heel and the other supporting the knee, bend the leg up to a 90-degree angle and rest the heel on the bed.

Stance   Walk-standing at ankle level.

Hands   One above the other on the back of the leg at ankle level with the elbows well away from the sides of the body.

One hand is moved firmly up the calf and, as it reaches to just below the knee, the other hand moves in the same way so that one hand is always moving and the other returning to the starting position. This can be repeated five or six times.

Return the leg to the lying position by supporting it at the knee and the heel.

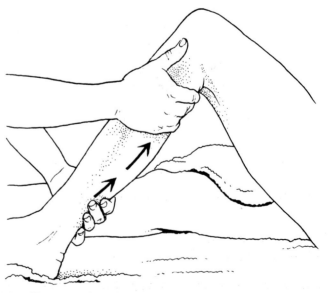

Figure 6.9 *Effleurage to the calf*

9 Effleurage to the lower leg

Stance   Walk-standing at level of the foot.

Hands   Cradling the foot as in the first effleurage movement.

Effleurage up the sides of the lower leg as far as the knee and return with a lighter stroking movement. Repeat two or three times.

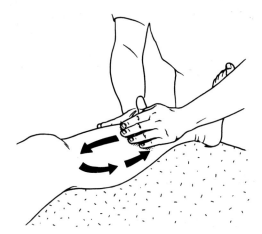

Figure 6.10 *Effleurage to the lower leg*

10 Thumb kneading to the anterior tibial muscles

Stance   Walk-standing at ankle level.

Hands   The working hand is placed on the outer side of the lower leg just below the knee with the other hand acting as a support on the inner surface.

The working hand kneads with the thumb in small circles down the outer surface to just above the ankle. Then the hand returns with an effleurage stroke to the beginning. Repeat once or twice.

> **REMEMBER**
> Avoid the anterior surface of the tibia, which is just under the skin.

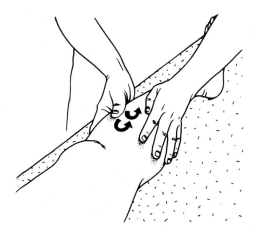

Figure 6.11 *Thumb kneading to the anterior tibial muscle*

11 Effleurage to the foot

Stance   Walk-standing below foot level.

Hands   One on the upper surface to support and the other, working hand, on the sole, both facing the same way.

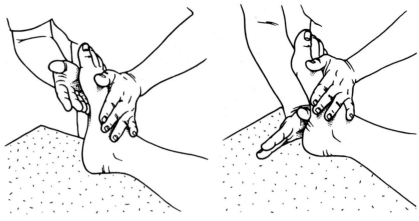

Figure 6.12 *Effleurage to the foot*

With the working hand fitting close into the sole of the foot, effleurage deeply from base of toes to the heel.

12 Kneading to the sole of the foot

Stance　Walk-standing below foot level.

Hands　One on the upper surface to support and the other, working hand, on the sole, both facing the same way.

Using the base of the thumb area to create pressure, perform circular kneading movements up and down the sole of the foot.

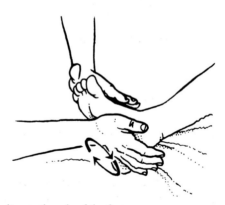

Figure 6.13 *Kneading to the sole of the foot*

13 Single-handed hacking to the sole of the foot

Stance　Walk-standing below foot level.

Hands　With one hand supporting the upper surface of the foot, use the other hand to lightly hack over the arched part of the sole.

14 Thumb stroking to the top of the foot

Stance　Walk-standing below foot level.

Hands　Fingers under the foot and the thumbs on top.

With the thumbs, stroke the top of the foot from the base of the toes upwards. The thumbs should stroke along the spaces between all the long metatarsal bones of the foot.

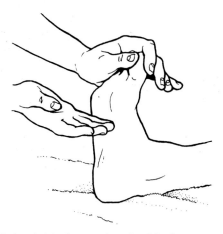

Figure 6.14 *Single-handed hacking to the sole of the foot*

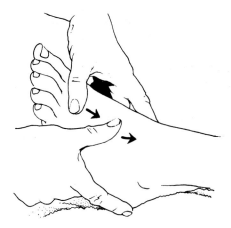

Figure 6.15 *Thumb stroking to the top of the foot*

15 Thumb stroking across the sole of the foot

Stance   Walk-standing below foot level.

Hands   Fingers on top of the foot and the thumbs under the foot lying across the sole.

Move the arms so that the thumbs move firmly across the sole of the foot crossing and uncrossing. Repeat the movement as the hands slide down from toes to heel.

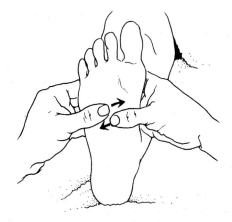

Figure 6.16 *Thumb stroking across the sole of the foot*

16 Kneading to the toes

Stance Walk-standing below foot level.

Hands Each toe in turn is grasped.

Each toe is gently grasped and rolled between the thumb and forefinger and at the same time gently pulled.

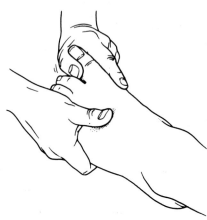

Figure 6.17 *Kneading to the toes*

17 Effleurage to the whole leg

Complete the leg massage by repeating the first effleurage strokes to the whole leg, to the front and to the sides. As these are the last movements before going on to the next part of the body they should get lighter and slower towards the end.

 Progress Check

Practise the leg massage until you can perform it fluently within 7 to 8 minutes.

Cover the right leg. Walk around the base of the couch to remove the covers from the left leg and proceed in exactly the same manner. Then proceed to the arm massage.

Arm massage (left)

Although the pattern of movements on the arm are similar to those on the leg, the technique needs to be different. The leg is a heavy limb which will stay in place as you carry out the manipulations whereas the arm is much lighter and not so densely covered in muscle.

There are a number of ways in which the arm can be supported during massage and as a therapist you will find your own preferred method. The arm may be supported by one of your hands and and rest along one arm while the other hand works, or the arm may lie on the bed while you use both hands to work. A mixture of these two methods will be described.

In general, the pattern of movements is similar in that effleurage movements start and finish the massage with petrissage and percussion in between.

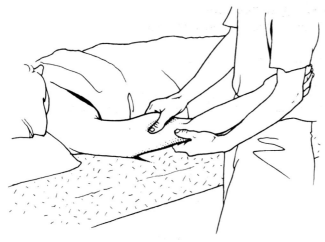

Figure 6.18 *Supporting the arm*

Superficial muscles

Deltoid

Pectoralist major

Biceps

Brachialis

Latissimus dorsi

Brachioradialis

Flexor carpi radialis

Palmaris longus

Flexor digitorum superficialis

Flexor carpi ulnaris

(Right arm)

Bones

Clavicle

Coracoid process

Acrominon process

Greater tubercle

Lesser tubercle

Scapula

Humerus

Medial epicondyle

Lateral epicondyle

Trochlea

Ulna

Radius

Carpal bones

Metacarpal bones

Phalanges

(Left arm)

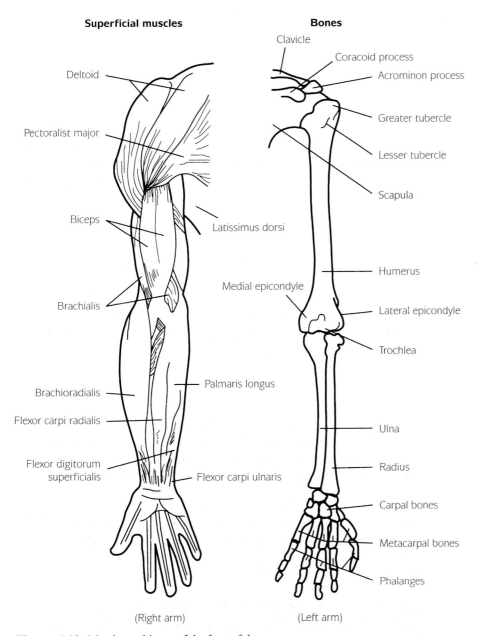

Figure 6.19 *Muscles and bones of the front of the arm*

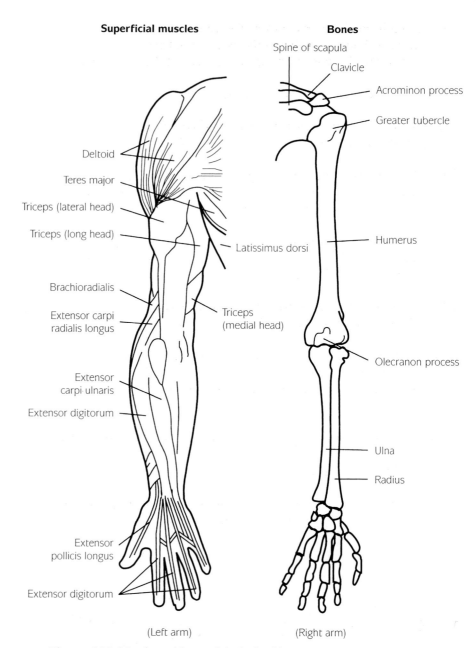

Superficial muscles

Deltoid

Teres major

Triceps (lateral head)

Triceps (long head)

Latissimus dorsi

Brachioradialis

Extensor carpi radialis longus

Triceps (medial head)

Extensor carpi ulnaris

Extensor digitorum

Extensor pollicis longus

Extensor digitorum

(Left arm)

Bones

Spine of scapula

Clavicle

Acrominon process

Greater tubercle

Humerus

Olecranon process

Ulna

Radius

(Right arm)

Figure 6.20 *Muscles and bones of the back of the arm*

The following are SUGGESTED MASSAGE MOVEMENTS for the arm.

1 Effleurage to the posterior aspect of the arm.
2 Effleurage to the anterior aspect of the arm.
3 Single-handed picking up to the deltoid and triceps muscles.
4 Single-handed picking up to the biceps muscle.
5 Wringing to the whole upper arm.
6 Light hacking to the upper arm.
7 Effleurage to the forearm.
8 Single-handed picking up to the forearm muscles.
9 Thumb stroking to the palm of the hand.
10 Thumb kneading to thenar (thumb) muscles and the hypothenar (little finger muscles).
11 Kneading to individual fingers and the thumb with stretching.

12 Thumb stroking to the back of the hand.
13 Circular thumb kneading to the back of the hand.
14 Repeat the effleurage to the front and back of the whole arm.

To start, fold back the towel to expose the arm.

1 Effleurage to the posterior aspect of the arm

Stance Walk-standing in the direction of the stroke.

Hands The left hand supports the upper arm near the axilla (armpit) so that the whole arm and hand of the client lies on the left arm of the therapist. This leaves the right hand free to work.

With the right hand moulded over the hand, effleurage up to and around the shoulder, returning to the hand with a lighter stroke. Repeat two or three times.

2 Effleurage to the anterior aspect of the arm

Stance Walk-standing in the direction of the stroke.

Hands The arm is turned to rest on the right hand and arm of the therapist whose left hand is now free to work. With the left hand moulded to the part, effleurage firmly up to the axilla and lightly down.

3 Single-handed picking up to the deltoid and triceps muscles

Stance Walk-standing in the direction of the stroke.

Hands As in movement 1, effleurage to the posterior aspect of the arm, so that the right hand is free to work and the arm is supported.

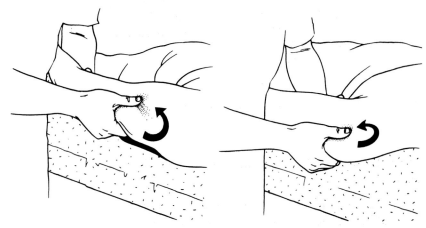

Figure 6.21 *Single-handed picking up of the deltoid and triceps muscles*

With the right hand moulded over the upper part of the deltoid muscle at the top of the arm, pick up the muscle from the bone, squeeze, release and move down a little. When the hand reaches the lower part of deltoid slide it back a little to cover the triceps muscle and pick up until the hand reaches a level of just above the elbow. Slide the hand up to reach the top of the arm and repeat a number of times.

REMEMBER
Don't dig in with the fingertips; there is no muscular covering to the sides of the upper arm.

4 Single-handed picking up of the biceps

Stance   Walk-standing in the direction of the stroke.

Hands   As in movement 2, effleurage to the anterior aspect of the arm, so that the client's arm is supported and your left hand is free to work.

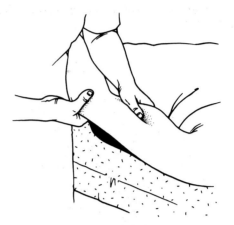

Figure 6.22 *Single-handed picking up of the biceps*

With the left hand moulded over biceps just below the axilla, pick up, squeeze and release, moving the hand down gradually until just above the elbow. Slide the hand firmly up to the top and repeat.

5 Wringing to the upper arm

The arm is placed on the pillow above the client's head for this movement.

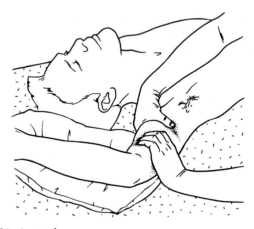

Figure 6.23 *Wringing to the upper arm*

Stance   Stride-standing to face across the client.

Hands   Both working, facing each other, with elbows well out to the sides.

Alternate hands lift the tissue, squeeze it and the fingers of one hand pull it towards you while the thumb of the other hand pushes it away. The hands wring up and down the upper arm to cover all the accessible muscle tissue.

6 Light hacking over the upper arm

The arm can be placed by the side of the body.

Stance   Stride-standing to face across the client.

Hands   Both working, with palms facing each other and elbows well out.

Lightly hack over the accessible muscle tissue using the outer surface of the little, ring and middle fingers only, not the border of the hand.

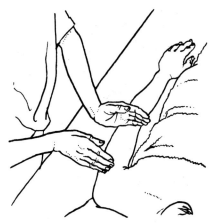

Figure 6.24 *Light hacking over the upper arm*

7 Effleurage to the forearm

Stance   Walk-standing facing the head of the couch.

Hands   The left hand holds the hand of the client so that the client's elbow is bent and resting on the couch.

With the right hand moulded around the forearm at wrist level, effleurage firmly down to the elbow, then stroke lightly up to repeat two or three times.

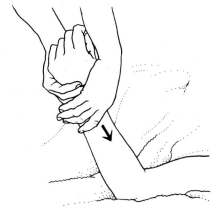

Figure 6.25 *Effleurage to the forearm*

8 Single-handed picking up to the forearm

Stance   Walk-standing facing the head of the couch.

Hands   The left hand holds the hand of the client so that the client's elbow is bent and resting on the couch.

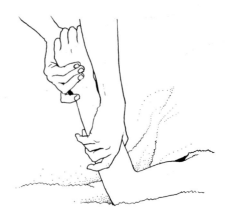

Figure 6.26 *Single-handed picking up of the forearm*

REMEMBER
Keep the palm of the working hand in contact as much as possible.

With the right hand moulded around the forearm at wrist level, pick up and release the tissue at the side of the forearm. Work towards the elbow, then back to the wrist, picking up the muscles on the front of the forearm.

9 Thumb stroking to the palm

Stance Walk-standing facing across the client.

Hands Hold the client's hand so that the elbow is slightly bent and resting on the bed. The therapist places one little finger between the thumb and forefinger of the client's hand so that the thumb is held out of the way and the other between the little finger and ring finger. The therapist's thumbs should now lie on the palm of the hand.

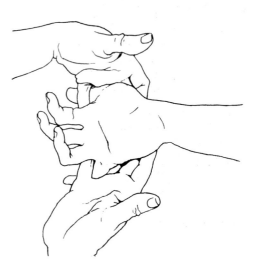

Figure 6.27 *Supporting the hand for thumb stroking and kneading to the palm*

With both thumbs, stroke the palms firmly from base of fingers to the wrist.

10 Thumb kneading to the thenar and hypothenar muscles

Stance Walk-standing facing across the client.

Hands As for movement 9, thumb stroking to the palm.

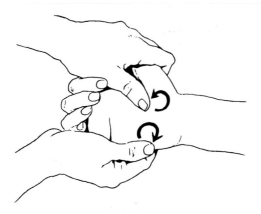

Figure 6.28 *Thumb kneading to the thenar and hypothenar muscles*

Both thumbs perform circular kneading movements over the muscular tissue.

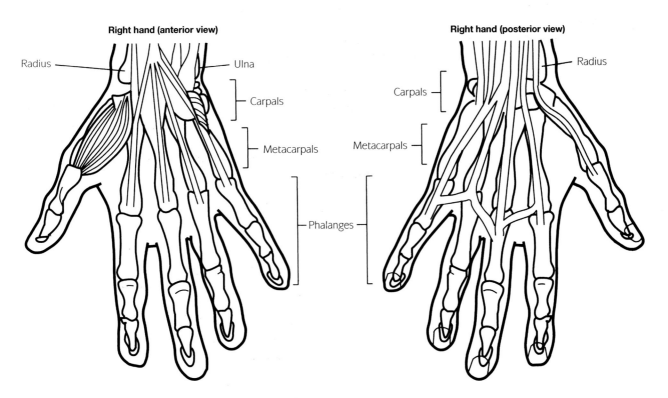

Right hand (anterior view)

Radius — — Ulna

Carpals

Metacarpals

Phalanges

Right hand (posterior view)

Radius

Carpals

Metacarpals

Figure 6.29 *Structure of the hand*

11 Kneading to individual fingers

Stance Walk-standing facing across the client.

Hands One hand supports the client's hand at the wrist.

Each finger is taken in turn and kneaded from base to tip between the fingers and thumb of the therapist. As each finger is completed, gentle traction is applied holding the whole finger along its length.

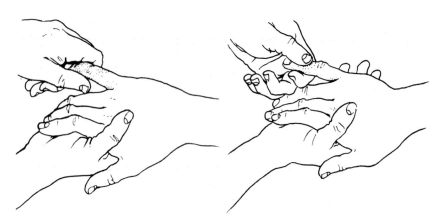

Figure 6.30 *Kneading to individual fingers*

12 Thumb stroking to the back of the hand

Stance Walk-standing facing across the client.

Hands Both supporting the client's hand with the back of the hand facing upwards.

       With the tips of the thumbs running between the metacarpal bones, stroke firmly up towards the wrist.

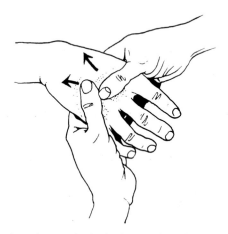

Figure 6.31 *Thumb stroking to the back of the hand*

13 Circular thumb kneading to the back of the hand

Stance Walk-standing facing across the client.

Hands As for movement 12, thumb stroking to the back of the hand.

       Taking care not to press too hard on the metacarpals, perform small circular kneading movements up and down the back of the hand with both thumbs.

14 Effleurage to the front and back of the whole arm

Repeat the effleurage movements to the whole arm as described in movements 1 and 2.

The arm should be placed under the towel before continuing the massage.

Practise the arm massage until it is fluent and can be performed within 5 to 6 minutes.

Chest massage

The preferred position for the therapist during this short part of the body massage is at the head of the bed. If this is not possible, then movements may be adapted to be performed from one side.

The towel covering the upper part of the body should be folded back to expose the upper chest and shoulders. This is also a good opportunity to remove any pillows from under the client's head, allowing greater access to the neck and shoulder region.

Care must be taken during massage to this area as the tissue is generally sensitive. Effleurage and suitable petrissage movements are used but rarely any percussion. Although this is a chest massage, the position of the body allows quite deep massage to the back of the neck and shoulders and these should be integrated into this part of the treatment.

> **ACTIVITY**
> Remind yourself of the arrangement of the bones and muscles of the chest and upper back.

Use the first effleurage strokes to apply the massage medium to the whole area.

The following are SUGGESTED MASSAGE MOVEMENTS for the chest.

1. Effleurage to the chest and the back of the neck with slight traction.
2. Stroking to one side of the neck with alternate hands.
3. Stroking to the other side of the neck with alternate hands.
4. Finger kneading to the upper fibres of the trapezius muscle from the shoulders to the base of the skull.
5. Kneading to the front of the chest and shoulders.
6. Effleurage to the chest and the back of the neck.

1 Effleurage to the chest and the back of the neck with slight traction

Stance Walk-standing at the head of the couch.

Hands Both hands are placed side by side on the sternum.

Stroke down the chest just far enough not to impinge on breast tissue, then, turning your hands to point outwards glide the hands over the chest towards the shoulders. The hands pass over the shoulders with the point of the shoulders fitting into the palms of the hands. With the hands in complete contact all the time, the fingers swivel towards each other onto the back of the

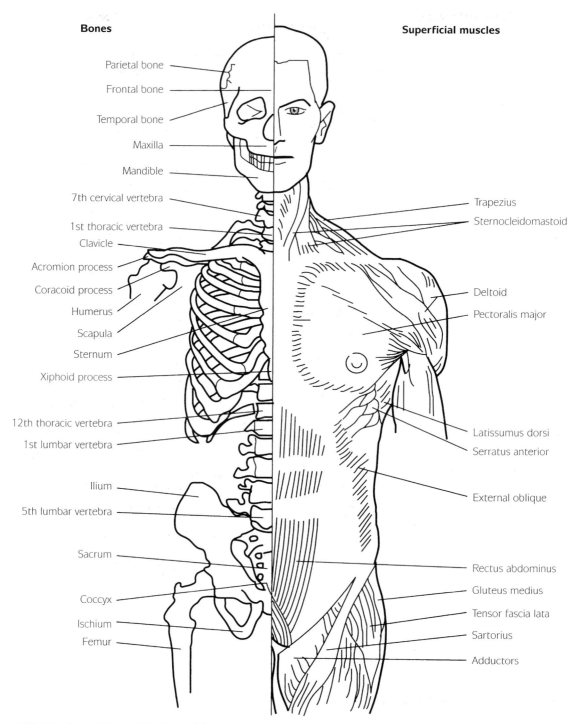

Bones

- Parietal bone
- Frontal bone
- Temporal bone
- Maxilla
- Mandible
- 7th cervical vertebra
- 1st thoracic vertebra
- Clavicle
- Acromion process
- Coracoid process
- Humerus
- Scapula
- Sternum
- Xiphoid process
- 12th thoracic vertebra
- 1st lumbar vertebra
- Ilium
- 5th lumbar vertebra
- Sacrum
- Coccyx
- Ischium
- Femur

Superficial muscles

- Trapezius
- Sternocleidomastoid
- Deltoid
- Pectoralis major
- Latissumus dorsi
- Serratus anterior
- External oblique
- Rectus abdominus
- Gluteus medius
- Tensor fascia lata
- Sartorius
- Adductors

Figure 6.32 *Muscles and bones of the front of the torso*

neck and stroke firmly upwards to the base of the skull. This must be done with a gentle pulling movement so that the head is not lifted off the bed. The hands return to the start with a light stroke down the side of the neck. Repeat four or five times

2 Stroking to one side of the neck with alternate hands

Stance Walk-standing at the head of the couch.

Hands One hand is cupped over the shoulder near the point of the shoulder.

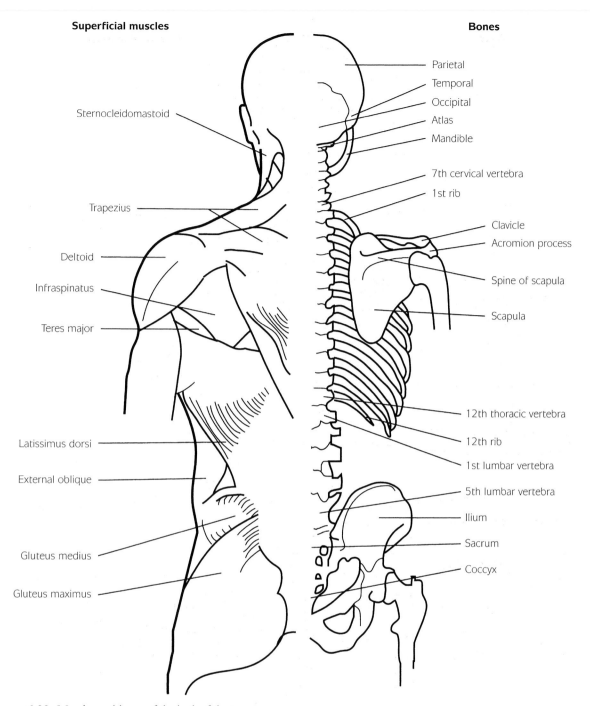

Figure 6.33 *Muscles and bones of the back of the torso*

Stroke firmly up the side of the neck to the base of the skull behind the ear, as it reaches the skull follow it with the other hand in exactly the same way. One of the hands should always be in contact as the other is returning to the start. The hands should be pointing down towards the bed during this movement and should be kept away from the front of the neck. Repeat several times.

3 Repeat stroking to the other side of the neck

Repeat the strokes of massage movement 2 on the other side of the neck.

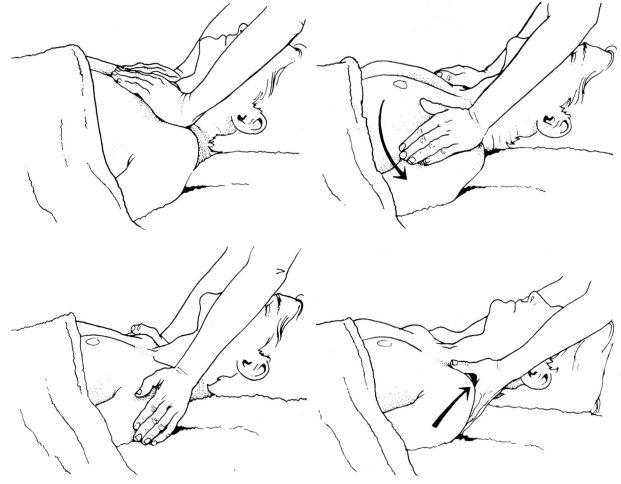

Figure 6.34 *Effleurage to the chest and back of the neck*

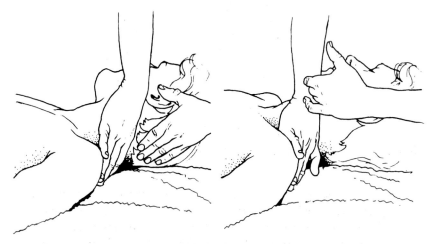

Figure 6.35 *Stroking to one side of the neck with alternate hands*

4 Finger kneading to the upper fibres of the trapezius

Stance   Walk-standing at the head of the couch.

Hands   Under the shoulders, palm up, with the fingertips on the muscle.

With both hands working, use the fingertips for firm, circular kneading movements along the muscle towards the centre then

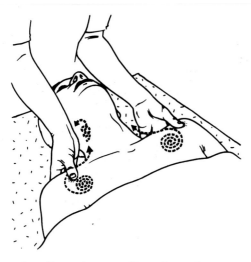

Figure 6.36 *Finger kneading to the upper fibres of trapezius*

up the back of the neck at the sides of the spine to the base of the skull. Slide the hands down to the start and repeat twice.

5 Kneading to the front of the chest and shoulders

Stance Walk-standing at the head of the couch.

Hands With hands lightly clenched, place the flat part of the fingers (between the knuckles and fingertips) on the centre of the chest side by side.

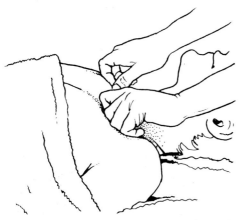

Figure 6.37 *Kneading to the front of the shoulders*

Using both hands, knead in circles very gently over the front of the chest moving outwards towards the shoulders. Move the hands, still kneading over the deltoid muscle then open the hands to sweep behind the shoulders and neck. Return to the start and repeat.

6 Effleurage to the chest and the back of the neck

Repeat the effleurage strokes of movement 1, but with less traction.

> **REMEMBER**
> When coming to the end of a massage to a particular area, the strokes should become lighter and slower.

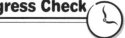

Progress Check

Practise until the chest massage can be completed fluently in 5 minutes.

Unfold the towel so that it covers the chest area and exposes the right arm.

Arm massage (right)

The massage strokes are a repeat of those used on the left arm though the therapist's working hand changes. For example, where the right hand previously supported the left arm while the left hand worked, now the left hand does the supporting while the right hand works.

Finish the arm by covering with the towel and expose the abdomen by folding back the upper and lower towels.

Abdomen massage

> **SAFE PRACTICE**
>
> The abdomen should be included in the body massage only if the therapist is sure that it is appropriate. The specific contraindication is pregnancy especially during the early months. In the last months of pregnancy, some gentle effleurage movements may be performed over the abdominal wall, but only after consultation with the client's medical advisors.

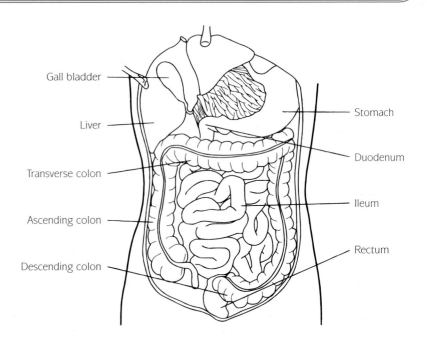

Figure 6.38 *Superficial structures of the abdomen*

> **REMEMBER**
> The abdominal organs will be affected by massage so the movements should not be too deep. Pressure over the bladder is uncomfortable and can be painful if the client has not been given the opportunity to empty the bladder before the massage.

Many female clients prefer not to have the abdomen worked over during their menstrual period and this should always be respected. Others look to a massage to relieve the discomfort felt in the first few days of menstruation and so long as the movements are gentle and the client warned that the menstrual flow may be increased, then there should be no problem.

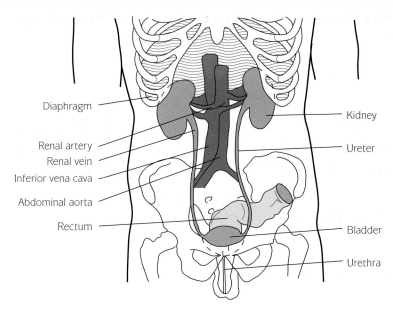

Diaphragm

Renal artery
Renal vein
Inferior vena cava
Abdominal aorta
Rectum

Kidney

Ureter

Bladder

Urethra

Figure 6.39 *Deep structures of the abdomen*

It is often helpful to place a rolled up towel or small pillow under the client's knees so that the abdominal wall is relaxed.

The following are SUGGESTED MASSAGE MOVEMENTS for the abdomen.

1 Effleurage to the abdomen.
2 Circular stroking to the abdomen.
3 Circular kneading over the colon.
4 Wringing to the sides and front of the abdomen.
5 Effleurage.

1 Effleurage to the abdomen

Stance Walk-standing close to the couch at the level of the client's hip.

Hands Placed side by side on the front of the abdomen above the pubis. Without applying much pressure, move the hands upwards until the fingers reach the bottom of the sternum, then turn the hands to point down towards the bed and continue to sweep down over the ribs, down the side of the waist, and then bring them up inside the iliac crest, wrists first, to the starting point. This is a very relaxing stroke and can be repeated four or five times increasing the pressure slightly.

2 Circular stroking to the abdomen

Stance Walk-standing close to the couch at the level of the client's hip.

Hands The main working hand is placed flat on the abdomen to one side just below the ribs with the other placed slightly behind it.

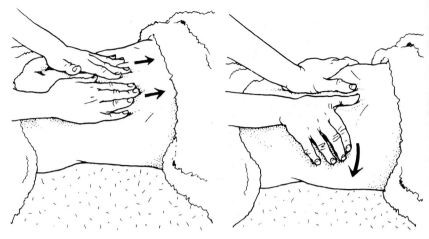

Figure 6.40 *Effleurage to the abdomen*

The first hand strokes in a large circle over the colon in a clockwise direction, up the right side, across the top and down the left side of the abdomen. This hand stays in contact all the time while circling. The other hand follows the main working hand but has to cross over the working hand to complete the circle.

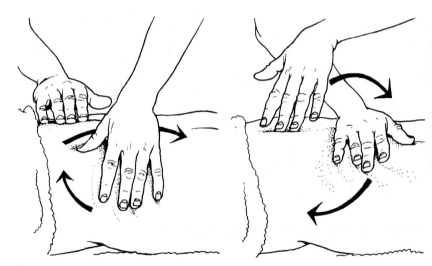

Figure 6.41 *Circular stroking to the abdomen*

3 Circular kneading over the colon

Stance   Walk-standing close to the couch at the level of the client's hip.

Hands   The main working hand is in the same starting position as for movement 2 and applies circular stroking to the abdomen, but with the other hand placed lightly on top.

Following the same clockwise direction, small circular kneading movements are performed over the colon.

4 Wringing to the sides and front of abdomen

Stance   Walk-standing facing across the client.

Hands   Placed facing each other on the far side of the waist. Pick up the tissue on the far side of the waist and wring up and down the

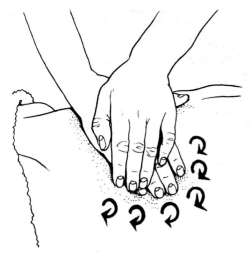

Figure 6.42 *Circular kneading over the colon*

waist, the front of the abdomen and the near side of the waist, repeating three or four times.

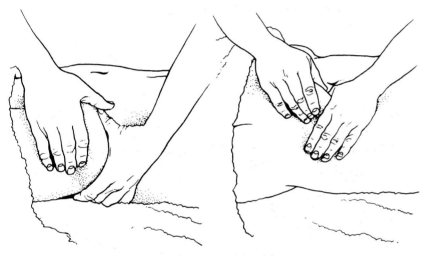

REMEMBER
Bend your knees to reach the near side of the waist.

Figure 6.43 *Wringing to the sides and front of the abdomen*

5 Effleurage to the abdomen

Repeat the first effleurage stroke four or five times. As this is the end of the massage to the front of the body, make the effleurage movements slower and slower and at the end, cup your hands over the navel. The warmth from your hands is a comforting end to this part of the massage.

Progress Check

Practise until you can perform the abdominal massage in 4 to 5 minutes.

Remove the rolled towel or pillow from under the knees and holding the towels in position, ask the client to turn over into the prone position. Any remaining pillows should be removed so that the head lies flat.

The back of the right leg (including buttock)

The lower towel is folded back to expose the whole of the leg and buttock region. It is usually of benefit to place a small rolled up towel under the ankle of the leg to be worked on. This helps the muscles on the back of the leg to relax and stops the foot being pressed onto the bed which would be uncomfortable.

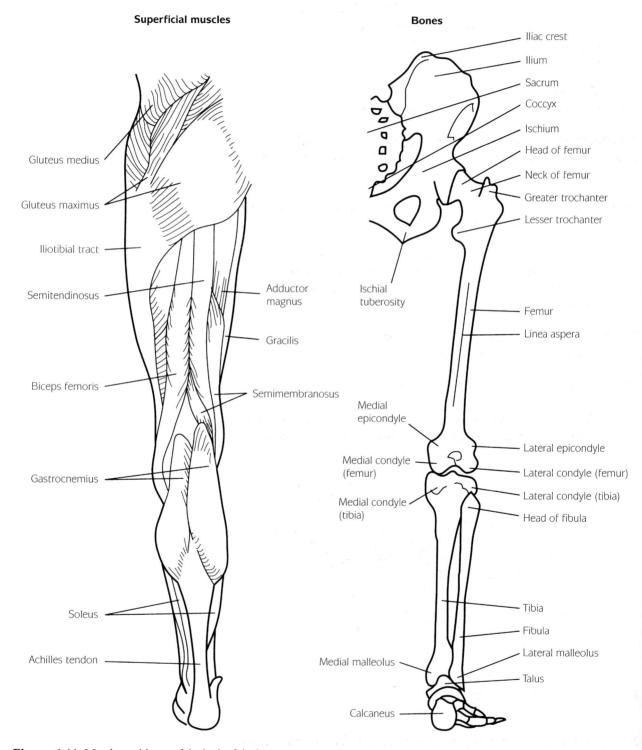

Superficial muscles

Gluteus medius

Gluteus maximus

Iliotibial tract

Semitendinosus

Biceps femoris

Gastrocnemius

Soleus

Achilles tendon

Adductor magnus

Gracilis

Semimembranosus

Bones

Iliac crest

Ilium

Sacrum

Coccyx

Ischium

Head of femur

Neck of femur

Greater trochanter

Lesser trochanter

Ischial tuberosity

Femur

Linea aspera

Medial epicondyle

Medial condyle (femur)

Medial condyle (tibia)

Lateral epicondyle

Lateral condyle (femur)

Lateral condyle (tibia)

Head of fibula

Medial malleolus

Tibia

Fibula

Lateral malleolus

Talus

Calcaneus

Figure 6.44 *Muscles and bones of the back of the leg*

The following are SUGGESTED MASSAGE MOVEMENTS for the back of the leg.

1. Effleurage to the back of the leg and the buttock.
2. Effleurage to the thigh and buttock.
3. Single-handed kneading to the outer surface of the thigh.
4. Reinforced kneading to the buttock and back of thigh.
5. Wringing over the buttock and back of thigh.
6. Double-handed picking up over the hamstring muscles.
7. Hacking over the buttocks and back of thigh.
8. Pounding or beating over the buttocks and back of thigh.
9. Clapping over the buttocks and back of thigh.
10. Effleurage to the buttock and thigh.
11. Effleurage to the calf.
12. Wringing to the calf muscles.
13. Light hacking to the calf.
14. Effleurage to the back of the leg and the buttock.

1 Effleurage to the back of the leg and the buttock

Stance Walk-standing at a level which allows the therapist to reach the whole length of the leg.

Hands The inner hand should be on the sole of the foot and the outer hand on the outer surface of the ankle.

Both hands effleurage firmly up the leg, over the buttock with the hands sweeping to the outer surface of the hip towards the groin to finish the stroke before returning to the start. Repeat four or five times.

2 Effleurage to the thigh and buttock

Stance Walk-standing at knee level.

Hands Placed one above the other above the knee across the thigh.

Sweep both hands up the thigh and over the buttocks where they separate and return to the start down the sides of the thigh.

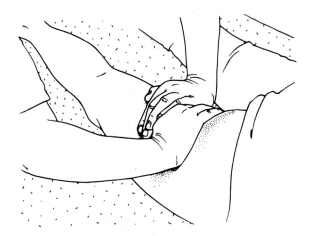

Figure 6.45 *Effleurage to the thigh and buttock*

3 Single-handed kneading to the outer surface of the thigh

Stance Walk-standing at knee level.

Hands The outer, working hand is placed on the outer surface of the hip and the inner hand rests and supports the thigh.

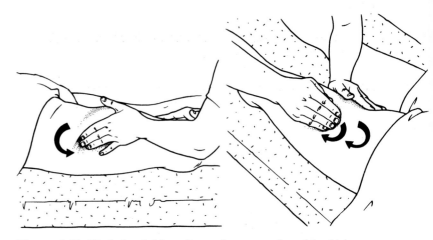

Figure 6.46 *Single-handed kneading to the outer surface of the thigh*

With the outer hand, knead in circles, moving gradually down the thigh to just above the knee. Then work in the same way up the thigh again.

4 Reinforced kneading to the buttock and back of thigh
Stance Walk-standing at knee level.

Hands The working hand is flat on the buttock, with the other hand resting on it.

With circular movements, knead over the buttock area taking care not to pull the buttocks apart, then down the back of the thigh to just above the knee. Use a sweeping effleurage stroke to return to the start. Repeat once.

5 Wringing to the buttock and back of thigh
Stance Walk- or stride-standing facing across the client.

Hands Placed on the inner thigh, just above the knee with fingers together and thumbs apart. Wring in the same way as on the

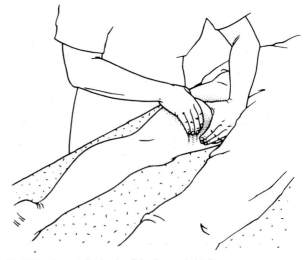

Figure 6.47 *Wringing to the back of the leg and thigh*

front of the leg, working up the thigh, over the buttock and down until the whole thigh and buttock is covered, repeat once or twice.

6 Double-handed picking up over the back of the thigh

Stance Walk-standing facing up the body.

Hands Placed high on the thigh forming a wide V-shape with the thumb of one hand alongside the index finger of the other hand.

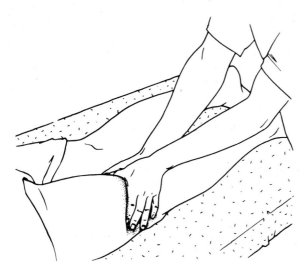

Figure 6.48 *Double-handed picking up over the back of the thigh*

Squeeze the muscles between both hands, lift and release and move the hands lower down. Repeat moving up and down the thigh covering the whole area two or three times.

7 Hacking to the buttocks and back of the thigh

Stance Walk- or stride-standing facing across the body.

Hands Relaxed and with the palms facing each other a little way apart and the elbows held well away from the sides.

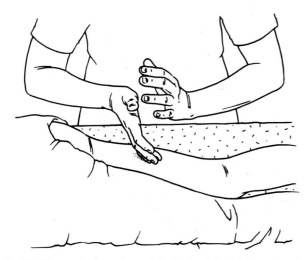

Figure 6.49 *Hacking to the buttocks and the back of the thigh*

Start hacking lightly down the back of the thigh and up again to cover the whole of the buttocks and back and outer surface of the thigh two or three times.

8 Pounding or beating over the buttocks and back of the thigh

Stance   Walk- or stride-standing facing across the body.

Hands   Lightly clenched, held side by side above the surface of the thigh. The wrists should be very loose. The part is struck with alternate hands using the ulnar side of the fist. Cover the part two or three times.

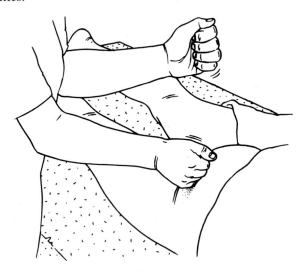

Figure 6.50 *Pounding over the buttocks and the back of the thigh*

9 Clapping over the buttocks and back of the thigh

Stance   Walk- or stride-standing facing across the body.

Hands   Cupped with fingers straight and thumbs close into the side of the fingers.

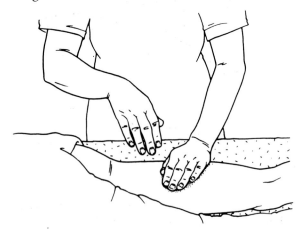

Figure 6.51 *Clapping over the buttocks and the back of the thigh*

The hands strike the part alternately, producing a dull hollow sound, not a slap. The whole of the back of the thigh and buttock may be covered once or twice.

10 Effleurage over the buttock and thigh
Repeat the strokes of movement 2.

11 Effleurage to the calf
Stance Walk-standing at the level of the ankle.

Hands One above the other, lying across the calf above the ankle.

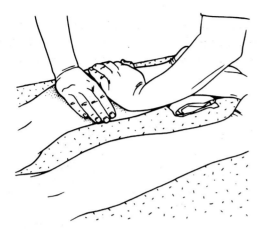

Figure 6.52 *Effleurage to the calf*

Both hands sweep upwards as far as the knee and separate for the return, downward strokes on the outer surfaces of the lower leg.

12 Wringing to the calf
Stance Stride-standing facing across the body.

Hands Placed on the calf, facing each other with the fingers together and thumbs apart.

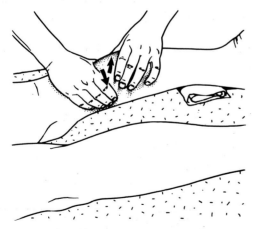

Figure 6.53 *Wringing to the calf*

Wring the calf muscles up and down between knee and ankle covering the whole area two or three times.

13 Light hacking to the calf
Stance Stride-standing facing across the body.

Hands Relaxed with palms facing each other alittle way apart and the elbows held well away from the sides.

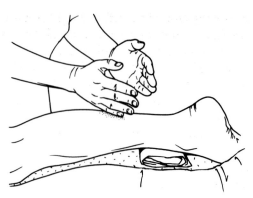

Figure 6.54 *Light hacking to the calf*

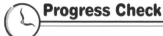

REMEMBER
If there is any evidence of varicose veins in the area, only light effleurage should be used over the calf.

Progress Check

Lightly hack up and down the calf covering the whole area two or three times

14 Effleurage to the back of the leg and the buttocks

Repeat the strokes of movement 1. As this is the last movement in this part of the massage, it should be performed so that the movements get slower and lighter towards the end.

Practise the massage to the back of the legs until it can be completed in 5 to 6 minutes.

When both legs are completed, cover the legs with towels, making sure that the feet are covered and fold down the top towel to expose the back from the shoulders to the level of the top of the sacrum.

Back massage

Look at figure 6.33 to remind yourself of the back's bones and muscles.

Very occasionally a client may benefit from a small pillow or folded towel under the abdomen during this part of the massage. For instance clients with a very hollow back or with large breasts will be able to lie prone with more comfort.

The client's hands may be placed under the forehead or at the sides. If they are under the forehead, the elbows should be quite low to allow the therapist to massage the shoulder area.

The back is the last part of the body to be massaged in this routine and, as such, is the part that will make the final impression on the client. The back is a large area with many bony points to be avoided or treated with care. The muscles tend to become very tense and should benefit a great deal from the massage.

The following are SUGGESTED MASSAGE MOVEMENTS for the back.

1 Reverse effleurage.
2 T-shaped effleurage.

3 Circular stroking around the left and right scapula.
4 Figure-of-eight reinforced stroking around the scapulae.
5 Flat-handed kneading to the whole back.
6 Single-handed picking up to the back of the neck.
7 Wringing to the shoulders and the tops of the arms.
8 Finger kneading/frictions at the sides of the spine.
9 T-shaped effleurage.
10 Effleurage towards the lymph nodes (lower cervical, axillary and inguinal)
11 Wringing to the sides of the back.
12 Skin rolling to the sides of the back.
13 Transverse stroking to the lumbar region.
14 Light hacking over the whole back.
15 T-shaped effleurage.

ACTIVITY

Before starting the back massage remind yourself of the bony points and the arrangement of the muscles.

1 Reverse effleurage

Stance Walk- or stride-standing at the head of the couch, standing close enough to the couch to be able to reach the whole length of the back.

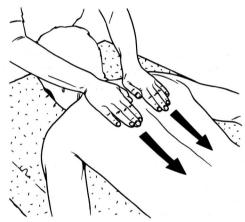

Figure 6.55 *Reverse effleurage*

Hands Placed flat on the upper back one on each side of the spine.

The hands are moved downwards to the base of the spine, then moved to the sides of the hips and glide firmly up the sides of the back to resume the starting position. The upward movement should be firmer than the downward one.

SAFE PRACTICE

Protect your back by not stretching further than you can easily reach. A short therapist may like to omit this movement.

Keeping one hand in contact with the body for the sake of continuity move around to the side of the couch.

2 T-shaped effleurage

Stance Walk-standing at a level allowing you to reach the whole length of the back. Choose the side of the couch which is best for you. A right-handed therapist will usually choose to work from the left side of the client.

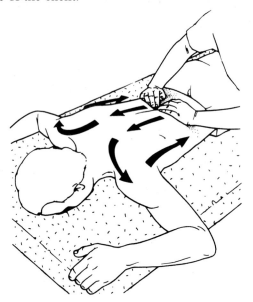

Figure 6.56 *T-shaped effleurage*

Hands Flat on the back at the base of the spine, one hand on each side of the spine.

Effleurage firmly up the sides of the spine to the base of the neck, slide outwards to the shoulders, over the upper arms, back to the shoulders and down the sides of the back to the start. The pressure should be greater on the upwards movement but the whole should be flowing and continuous.

3 Circular stroking around the left and right scapula

Stance Walk-standing at waist level.

Hands The main working hand is placed flat between the scapulae with the other slightly behind it. In this movement, the hands circle the scapula in an upwards and outwards direction. Thus, the right scapula is circled in a clockwise direction and the left in an anticlockwise direction.

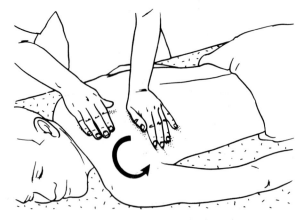

Figure 6.57 *Circular stroking around the left scapula*

The main working hand circles the scapula and remains in contact, the other hand follows but has to be lifted to pass over the main working hand at each circle. This can be done four or five times around one scapula then the same around the other.

4 Figure-of-eight reinforced stroking around the scapulae

Stance Walk-standing at waist level.

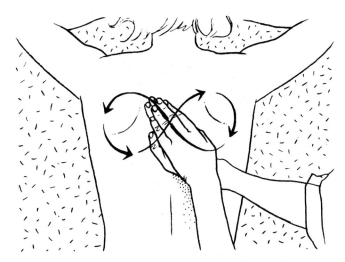

Figure 6.58 *Figure-of-eight reinforced stroking around the scapulae*

Hands The main working hand is placed between the scapulae with the other hand on top of it.

Move the hands upwards between the scapulae, around one scapula then the other in a figure-of-eight. The pressure should be deeper on the upward part of the movement.

5 Flat-handed kneading

Stance Walk-standing at a level to be able to reach the whole back.

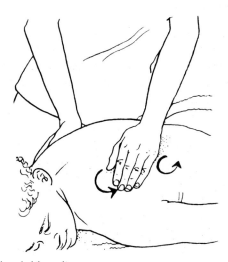

Figure 6.59 *Flat-handed kneading*

Hands The working hand is flat on the upper back with the other hand resting on the other side.

Knead in circles with the hand flat on the skin moving the superficial tissues on deeper tissues and only moving over the skin to shift the position of the hands. Work down one side of the body and effleurage up to start again. Repeat on other side.

6 Single-handed picking up to the back of the neck

Stance Walk-standing just below shoulder level facing the head of the couch.

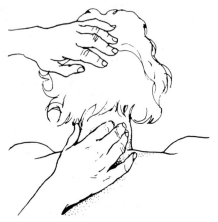

Figure 6.60 *Single-handed picking up to the back of the neck*

Hands The working hand is placed on the back of the neck, the other hand resting on the shoulder or the back of the head.

With the fingers and thumb spread, pick up the muscle mass at the base of the neck, squeeze and release. Move up to the base of the skull and down again.

7 Wringing to the shoulders and the tops of the arms

Stance Walk-standing just below shoulder level facing the head of the couch.

Hands Both lying on the curve of the neck with fingers and thumbs spread to grasp the muscle tissue.

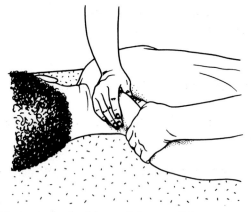

Figure 6.61 *Wringing to the shoulders and the tops of the arms*

Pick up and wring down the neck, across to the point of the shoulder and down over the upper arm. Continue picking up and move back up the arm, across to the neck, and then across the other shoulder and upper arm.

8 Finger kneading/frictions at the sides of the spine

Stance Walk-standing at waist level level facing the head of the couch.

Hands The tips of the middle fingers are placed on one side of the spine at the level of the base of the neck.

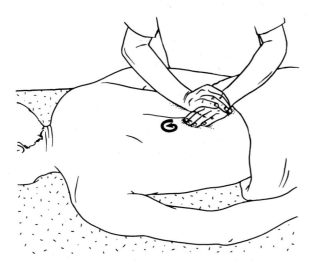

Figure 6.62 *Finger kneading/frictions at the side of the spine*

With the working fingers straight, feel for the slight hollows between the bony transverse processes of the vertebrae. Working downwards, knead with the fingertips in a circular direction in each hollow until the base of the spine is reached. This should be performed only once and the depth of the strokes depends on the physical state of the client. With someone young and fit, the movement may be deep enough to be considered as frictions. Repeat on the other side.

9 T-shaped effleurage to the whole back

Repeat the strokes of movement 2.

10 Effleurage towards the lymph nodes (lower cervical, axillary and inguinal)

Stance Walk-standing at a level allowing you to reach the whole length of the back.

Hands Flat on the back at the base of the spine, one hand on each side of the spine.

In the first effleurage stroke, the hands pass from the base of the back up over the back on either side of the spine to the shoulders and return to the base of the spine with a lighter pressure. The second stroke goes up the back and outwards to the axilla. The third up and out to the sides of the waist. This group of three movements may be repeated.

11 Wringing to the sides of the back

Stance Walk-standing facing across the client.

Hands Flat on the side of the waist furthest from the therapist.

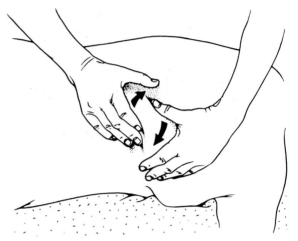

Figure 6.63 *Wringing to the sides of the back*

Wring down over the hip and up to the axilla. This can be repeated before moving the hands to the near side to wring in the same way.

12 Skin rolling to the sides of the back

Stance Walk-standing facing across the client.

Hands Flat on the side of the back furthest from the therapist with the fingers straight and the thumbs as far away from the fingers as possible. The thumb tips should be touching.

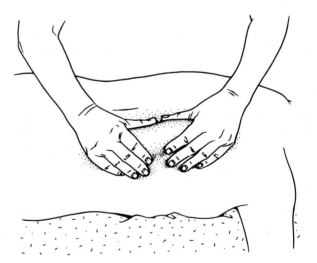

Figure 6.64 *Skin rolling to the sides of the back*

> **REMEMBER**
> To work on the near side, you must either turn your arms or reverse the use of the thumbs and fingers.

With the fingers flat, pull the skin upwards, then push the resulting roll of skin away towards the fingers with the long surface of the thumbs. The hands travel up and down the side of the body before moving to work on the other side.

13 Transverse stroking to the lumbar region

Stance Walk-standing facing across the client.

Hands Flat on the lower back.

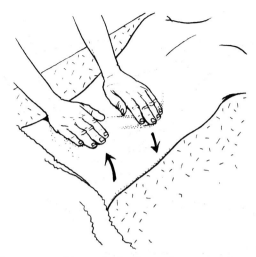

Figure 6.65 *Transverse stroking to the lumbar region*

With alternate hands, stroke across the lower back from the centre to the far side of the back, then from the centre to the near side. Repeat a number of times to cover the whole lumbar area.

14 Light hacking over the whole back

Stance Walk- or stride-standing facing across the back.

Hands Palms facing each other a little way apart and the elbows held well away from the sides.

Lightly hack up and down the whole length of the back remembering to avoid the bony points of the spine and scapula.

> **REMEMBER**
> The side of the hand is not used, only the sides of the fingers. The elbows should be well away from the sides.

15 T-shaped effleurage

Repeat the strokes of movement 2. This is the last movement of the whole massage. As it is repeated, the pace gets slower and the depth lighter until the last movement finishes with the hands lightly cupped over the base of the spine. Rest the hands for a moment or two before covering the back with the towels.

Clients should be left quietly for a little while at the end of a massage especially if the main aim of the massage is to induce relaxation. They may even be asleep. After a few minutes the client can be gently roused and asked if they want the massage medium, oil or cream removed from the skin. If so, this can be blotted off with tissue or gently wiped with cotton wool and a good cologne or cleansing cream.

When dressed, the client may be questioned as to the effectiveness of the treatment and the consultation card filled in as necessary before payment is taken and a further appointment offered.

Try a full body massage attempting to keep within one hour for the treatment.

Full body massage – summary

Front of legs

1 Effleurage to the sides and front of the whole of the leg.
2 Effleurage to the thigh.
3 Double-handed kneading to the thigh.
4 Single-handed kneading to the thigh.
5 Wringing to the thigh muscles.
6 Hacking to the thigh muscles.
7 Stroking around the knee.
8 Effleurage to the back of the calf with knee bent.
9 Effleurage to the lower leg.
10 Thumb kneading to the anterior tibial muscles.
11 Effleurage to the foot.
12 Kneading to the sole of the foot.
13 Single-handed hacking to the sole of the foot.
14 Thumb stroking to the top of the foot.
15 Thumb stroking across the sole of the foot.
16 Kneading to the toes.
17 Repeat of effleurage to the front and sides of the whole leg.

Arm massage

1 Effleurage to the posterior aspect of the arm.
2 Effleurage to the anterior aspect of the arm.
3 Single-handed picking up to the deltoid and triceps muscles.
4 Single-handed picking up to the biceps muscle.
5 Wringing to the whole upper arm.
6 Light hacking to the upper arm.
7 Effleurage to the forearm.
8 Single-handed picking up to the forearm muscles.
9 Thumb stroking to the palm of the hand.
10 Thumb kneading to the thenar (thumb) muscles and the hypothenar (little finger) muscles.
11 Kneading to individual fingers and the thumb with stretching.
12 Thumb stroking to the back of the hand.
13 Circular thumb kneading to the back of the hand.
14 Repeat the effleurage to the front and back of the whole arm.

Chest massage

1 Effleurage to the chest and the back of the neck with slight traction.
2 Stroking to one side of the neck with alternate hands.
3 Stroking to the other side of the neck with alternate hands.
4 Finger kneading to the upper fibres of the trapezius muscle from the shoulders to the base of the skull.
5 Kneading to the front of the chest and shoulders.
6 Effleurage to the chest and the back of the neck.

Abdomen

1 Effleurage to the abdomen.
2 Circular stroking to the abdomen.
3 Circular kneading over the colon.
4 Wringing to the sides and front of the abdomen.
5 Effleurage.

Back of leg

1 Effleurage to the back of the leg and the buttock.
2 Effleurage to the thigh and buttock.
3 Single-handed kneading to the outer surface of the thigh.
4 Reinforced kneading to the buttock and the back of the thigh.
5 Wringing over the buttock and back of the thigh.
6 Double-handed picking up over the hamstring muscles.
7 Hacking over the buttocks and the back of the thigh.
8 Pounding or beating over the buttocks and the back of the thigh.
9 Clapping over the buttocks and the back of the thigh.
10 Effleurage to the buttock and thigh.
11 Effleurage to the calf.
12 Wringing to the calf muscles.
13 Light hacking to the calf.
14 Effleurage to the back of the leg and the buttock.

Back

1 Reverse effleurage.
2 T-shaped effleurage.
3 Circular stroking around the left and right scapula.
4 Figure-of-eight reinforced stroking around the scapulae.
5 Flat-handed kneading to the whole back.
6 Single-handed picking up to back of neck.
7 Wringing to the shoulders and the tops of the arms.
8 Finger kneading/frictions at the sides of the spine.
9 T-shaped effleurage.
10 Effleurage towards the lymph nodes (lower cervical, axillary and inguinal).
11 Wringing to the sides of the back.
12 Skin rolling to the sides of the back.
13 Transverse stroking to the lumbar region.
14 Light hacking over the whole back.
15 T-shaped effleurage.

ACTIVITY

Start a diary to keep a record of all the massage clients you see and practise on. Note the details of their consultation and any information about their physical condition you gain during the massage.

ADAPTATIONS TO THE MASSAGE ROUTINE

After working through this chapter you will be able to:

♦ adapt the massage routine to individual areas of the body

♦ adapt the basic strokes to suit a variety of clients, thin/fat, male/female, young/old, fit/unfit

♦ adapt a body massage for a pregnant client

♦ demonstrate massage of small children or babies

♦ adapt massage to suit a number of disabilities

♦ adapt massage to suit a slimming programme

♦ outline the principles of lymphatic drainage massage

♦ outline the principles of massage to suit clients involved in sporting activities.

Massage to individual areas of the body

When clients do not wish for a whole body massage, it is quite usual to carry out massage to individual parts of the body. Sometimes massage is carried out as part of another treatment such as foot massage during a pedicure, hand massage during a manicure or chest or neck massage as part of a facial treatment. Sometimes a client may require massage to a particular area as a treatment in itself. If someone is unwell , a hand or foot massage may be all that is possible. This is particularly so when applying an aromatherapy massage in a hospital or hospice setting. The most common area to be massaged on its own is the back and shoulder when a client complains of tension and stiffness.

Back and shoulder massage
Timing
This may be from 15 to 30 minutes depending on the client's wishes.

Position
The client can take up a position of prone lying with the clothing removed from the upper part of the body as far as the buttocks.

The massage strokes may be the same as those described for the back in the general body massage, but more time can be allotted to the area, especially those parts, usually around the scapulae, which are tense and stiff. Thus after the figure-of-eight reinforced stroking, finger kneading movements around the scapulae may be performed. It is not unusual to feel 'nodules' of tension in the muscles here and in the shoulders and while it is important not to cause pain to the client, these may be worked on quite deeply. If this is the case the client should be warned of the tenderness that might be present afterwards.

It is not always necessary for the client to lie down for a back massage particularly if the shoulder area is the important part. The client may sit with the head resting on a table with a pillow or cushion as a support. If treating someone at home the client may sit astride a chair using the back of the chair as a support for the head. The arms may be under the forehead or resting on the knees, whichever is most comfortable.

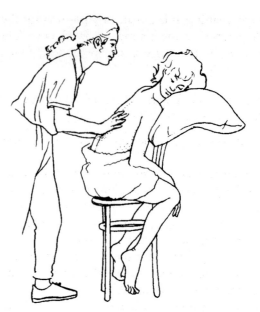

Figure 7.1 *Back massage in a sitting position using a kitchen chair*

There are specific supports on the market (see page 9, chapter 2) which can be placed on a table or couch for the client to rest on or be a complete support chair in itself. These are also convenient to use if you are visiting clients in the home or office.

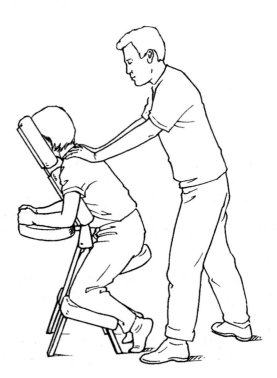

Figure 7.2 *Seated massage chair*

There has been a recent development in employers encouraging employees who are sitting for much of the working day, to receive on-site massage, often without leaving their workstations. In this case, the client retains their clothing and the massage is adapted by concentrating more on pressure and petrissage techniques.

When the client is sitting, it is not an easy position for the therapist and it takes a little practice for the massage to be effective. The position is suitable only for a short massage, as the lower half of the back cannot be worked on effectively.

The following is a SUGGESTED ROUTINE for back and shoulder massage if the client is in prone lying.

1 Effleurage to the upper back and shoulders and the tops of the arms.
2 Circular stroking around the right and left scapula.
3 Figure-of-eight reinforced stroking around the scapulae.
4 Flat-handed kneading over the upper back and shoulders.
5 Single-handed picking up to the back of the neck.
6 Wringing across the shoulders and the tops of the arms.
7 Finger kneading/frictions at the sides of the spine.
8 Finger kneading/frictions around the right and left scapula.
9 Light hacking across the shoulders.
10 Effleurage to the upper back and shoulders and the tops of the arms.

Foot and leg massage

This is often suggested for a client with tired feet or tired 'puffy' legs, for instance for a client who does a lot of standing rather than walking during the working day. (For lymphatic drainage massage see page 138.)

SAFE PRACTICE

Remember the contraindications to massage that might cause swelling of a limb are thrombosis, phlebitis or severe varicose veins. If in doubt, refer the client to their medical advisor, and never massage over tender or swollen areas when the cause is unknown.

Position

The client should be lying, and it will help the massage to be effective if the legs can be slightly elevated. This elevation can be achieved either by raising the end of the couch or by placing pillows under the whole length of the legs. The legs must not be raised more than about 25 degrees. At this angle lymphatic drainage can occur freely to the inguinal lymph nodes and massage is easy to apply. The legs should never be raised so high as to make the massage awkward for the therapist.

Preparation

The soles of the feet should be lightly wiped with cologne to remove any dirt or perspiration. The leg not being worked on should be covered with a towel.

The following is a SUGGESTED ROUTINE for foot and leg massage (the numbers of repetitions of each stroke depends on the time available).

1 Effleurage to the sides of the leg starting at the toes and ending at the inguinal nodes.
2 Effleurage to the sides of the lower leg and the front of the thigh.
3 Effleurage to the sides of the lower leg and the back of the thigh.
4 Double-handed circular kneading to the thigh.
5 Wringing to the thigh muscles.
6 Hacking to the thigh muscles.
7 Light beating or pounding to the thigh muscles.

8   Effleurage to the thigh.
9   Stroking around the knee.
10 Effleurage to the lower leg directed to the back of the knee.
11 With the leg rolled outwards, wringing to the calf muscles.
12 Effleurage to the lower leg.
13 Effleurage to the sole of the foot.
14 Kneading to the sole of the foot.
15 Single-handed hacking to the sole of the foot.
16 Thumb stroking to the top of the foot.
17 Thumb stroking across the sole of the foot.
18 Kneading with gentle traction to individual toes.
19 Effleurage to the whole leg.

The movements described for the hands and feet may be used on their own for a client who is bed-bound, for example a hospitalised patient.

When performing a leg and foot massage it may be appropriate to include some reflexology techniques as described in chapter 8.

 Progress Check

From the whole body massage routine, select movements suitable to make up:

a)   a hand massage routine
b)   a foot massage routine.

Carry out one of each.

Adapting massage to various clients

Adaptations to general massage should be made to accommodate clients of different age groups, sizes and physical and mental states.

The initial consultation procedure should elicit information useful for selecting massage movements and methods to suit individual clients. Information such as age, lifestyle and medical history can be gained in this way, but it is only when starting to massage that many physical characteristics are noted.

Client preference as to depth of massage should be obtained by direct questioning during the first treatment and noted on the treatment card for future reference. Often a client needs to be encouraged to give direction in this. It is not enough to ask, 'Is that alright?' or to say, 'Tell me if it is too deep'. The client needs to be told that it will help you if they can give a definite indication as to how firm they like the massage.

The muscle tone of a client can be felt when massage is being performed on the larger muscle groups and, in general, muscle tone is better in younger, fitter clients than in older ones. If muscle tone is poor then care must be taken with the petrissage and percussion movements so that the muscles are not compressed too hard against bone or overstretched during wringing or rolling techniques. Similar care must be taken with very thin clients, young or old, as deep massage over bony points will be very uncomfortable.

An obese client presents different problems. The muscle tone often cannot be easily assessed due to overlying fatty tissue and there may be a temptation to think that the density of the tissue means that it is insensitive. It is not unusual for an obese client to complain that massage is painful over areas such as the thighs. Client feedback must be obtained and noted.

In general terms, the male body is firmer than the female, although this depends on their fitness and exercise regime. Women have a layer of fat under the skin which softens the line of the female body, hiding the muscle outlines and making the body softer to handle.

The male body may be hairy which makes massage difficult. Hairy chests and legs are common but backs and arms can also be very hairy. If the body is hairy, then the massage must be adapted to avoid working against the lie of the hair.

- Use more oil or talc than usual to allow free movement of hands.
- Effleurage or stroking should be performed in the direction of the hair.
- When using petrissage, take care not to pull on the hair.

Clients book massage treatments for different reasons: for relaxation, for stimulation or alongside a slimming/fitness regime and this will also affect the type of massage given.

It should also be noted that many clients will be nervous at their initial treatments and it is the therapist's responsibility to put them at ease. An atmosphere of quiet and reassurance that professional standards are maintained is essential.

ACTIVITY
Try to select as wide a variety of clients as possible and in your massage diary note adaptations appropiate to age differences, size, fitness, etc.

Massage for the pregnant client

You should ask a pregnant client to check with her medical advisor whether there is any reason why she should not have massage.

Remember that massage over the abdomen is contraindicated during the first three months of a pregnancy.

Pregnant women often benefit from massage because they tend to tire more easily. Their posture alters as their figure shape changes, causing stress on the lower back and legs, and their weight increases causing tired legs and feet. Pregnant women often find sleep difficult and the relaxing effects of massage can help this insomnia.

A bland oil or cream may be used for the massage which will help the skin to stretch more easily over the abdomen. No essential oils should be used in the first three months of pregnancy and great care taken in the choice of oils later as many essential oils are contraindicated.

The body massage routine may be used with a number of adaptations.

- Omit any percussion/tapotement movements.
- All the movements should be smooth and gentle.
- The positioning of the client will need to be altered as she will be unable to lie on her stomach. For massage to the back and back of the legs, she can lie in the recovery position or on her side with supporting pillows under the upper leg and arm. When she lies on her back, put a small cushion under her knees to relax the abdomen and flatten the lower back.

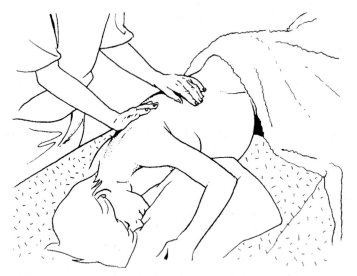

Figure 7.3 *Positioning a pregnant client for a massage to the back/back of legs*

The only movements that may be done over the abdomen (after three months) are stroking movements.

1   Stroke around the abdomen clockwise, using both hands, one following the other in a gentle flowing movement.
2   Stroke up the centre of the abdomen very gently and then very lightly down the sides.

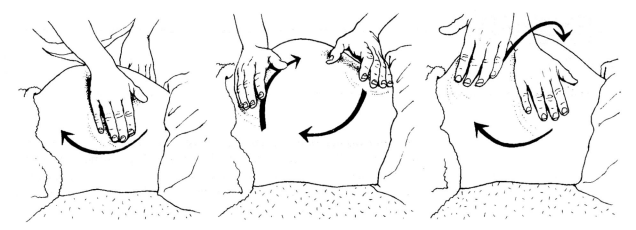

Figure 7.4 *Stroking on the abdomen of a pregnant client*

Children and babies

These are unlikely to be clients in a salon, but parents who benefit from massage will often ask how they can massage their children and you may find it a good idea to hold occasional classes for parents.

Baby massage classes:

- give the mother the opportunity to meet other parents and discuss problems
- promote bonding between parent and baby
- give the parent time for relaxation
- promote confidence in handling the baby.

The room should be warm, and relaxing music has been found to be useful for both babies and parents. Very often, the parents just require the confidence to try massage and a class with other parents is just the place to start.

Parents should be warned that children love to be massaged and they could find themselves still being asked for a massage when their children are grown up!

Babies

Babies love to be stroked and caressed and a loving touch is a natural part of parenting. Massage is just an extension of this which will benefit parent and baby by helping in the bonding process.

In many parts of the world, babies are massaged and rubbed from birth, sometimes even with the aim of moulding the shape of the head and body after a difficult birth.

Massage can help to calm a fractious baby and is of special benefit to parents who find they have a baby who is reluctant to sleep. It can calm the baby and the parent. The best time of day is just before or after the baby's bath. A tiny baby can be massaged lying along the parent's knee or on the changing table or floor, wherever is comfortable and convenient and eye contact can be encouraged.

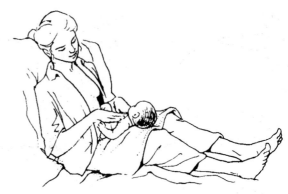

Figure 7.5 *Massaging a baby lying along the knees*

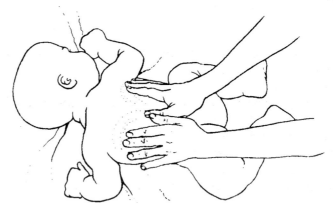

Figure 7.6 *Massaging a baby on a table or floor*

The massage medium should be a good quality vegetable oil, such as grapeseed or sunflower oil but preferably not baby oil as that is a mineral oil. It is probably wise to avoid nut oils especially peanut oil in case of allergy. If essential oils are to be added to the massage oil, they should be very dilute and care taken that there are no contraindications. Whichever massage oil is used, it should be light, not thick and should be slightly warmed before application. Talc is not suitable as the powder may be inhaled by the baby.

There is no need for a rigid or special sequence, the movements are nearly all stroking movements except for gentle squeezing and wringing with the fingertips on the limbs and back if the baby seems to enjoy it.

It's usual to start on the front of the baby's body so that they can see the parent.

The face can be included with gentle thumb stroking across the forehead centre to sides and around the nose and chin.

Babies, like adults, appear to prefer firm movements rather than light, tickly ones. Ten minutes for a baby massage is probably enough.

The following is a TYPICAL SEQUENCE for a baby masssage.

Start with the baby on its back.

1 Stroking the top of the head gently with the palm.
2 Stroking down the sides of the face from the crown of the head.

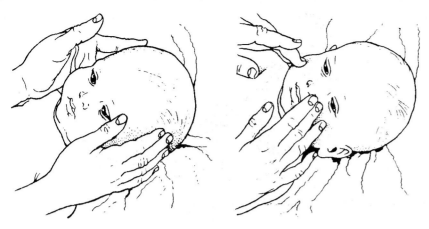

Figure 7.7 *Massaging a baby's face*

3 Gentle thumb stroking across the forehead, centre to sides and around the nose and chin.
4 Stroking down the arms and hands.
5 Gentle squeezing down each arm with the palm of the hand.
6 Circular stroking to the palms and backs of hands.
7 Stroking down the chest and abdomen.
8 Stroking down the legs and feet.
9 Circular stroking to the soles of the feet.
10 Stroking down the length of the body, neck to toes.

Turn the baby into a prone lying position.

1 Stroke down the back of the head and neck.
2 Make long strokes down the length of the back, from the neck to the base of the buttocks.
3 Make long strokes to the backs of the legs.
4 Make long strokes over body and legs.

Children

In the same way, clients who come for massage and express an interest can be encouraged to massage their children. Children of all ages enjoy it and respond well to relaxing strokes. It need not be a formal massage session, just some of the effleurage and petrissage strokes that are used on adults, but applied more lightly and for less time.

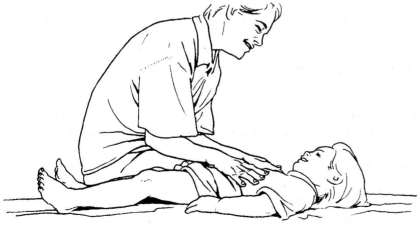

Figure 7.8 *Massaging children*

If a child becomes restless, that is the time to stop. There is often no need for the child to undress and have oil on the skin; massage can take place through light clothing and be part of a play session.

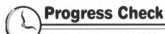

If you have access to a baby or young child in the family, try a short massage during their bathtime routine.

Massage for disabled clients

Massage is now becoming used as a therapy in the care of many groups with physical and mental problems. Treatment usually takes place within a hospital or other care setting and therapists will be guided by medical and nursing staff.

Uses of massage in hospital or other care settings

- To reduce pain and oedema.
- To reduce muscle tone and tension.
- To reduce stress and anxiety.
- To prevent pressure sores.
- To reduce constipation.
- To improve body image.
- To help communication.
- To develop sensory awareness.

Massage with essential oils is being used to great effect with clients who have learning difficulties, particularly when there are associated physical difficulties such as deafness or blindness.

In the same way, elderly patients with dementia benefit from massage, aromatherapy and the use of passive movements to help maintain mobility. Well-chosen essential oils can help insomnia. Psychologically, the pleasant aromas of oils can evoke memories and help to overcome institutional smells and associations. Essential oils are often burned or diffused into the atmosphere with similar results.

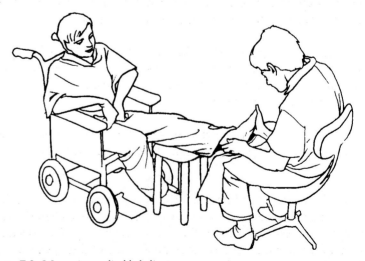

Figure 7.9 *Massaging a disabled client*

In salons or clinics, clients with a physical condition that affects movement can usually receive massage to suit them. A variable-height couch which is hydraulically or electronically controlled allows clients to reach the couch and then be raised to a height to suit the therapist.

A client who uses a wheelchair may transfer to a couch or prefer to be treated in the wheelchair.

If a request for treatment is made by someone with a neurological condition such as multiple sclerosis (MS) or by someone who has had a stroke or other serious illness, always consult their doctor.

Arthritis and rheumatic conditions sometimes limit clients' mobility and often cause pain in joints and the surrounding muscles.

SAFE PRACTICE

Remember that working over hot swollen joints is contraindicated.

Be guided by the client as to what position they can adopt. Then the massage can be adapted to suit that position. Pillows can be placed to support the body as necessary.

Avoid percussion/tapotement movements and be guided by the client when working on muscles near affected joints. Never work over painful areas.

You might find that you can work in conjunction with other therapists, perhaps the client's physiotherapist, to the advantage of you both. The physiotherapist will probably be concentrating on rehabilitation and maintaining normal movement and might welcome the help of someone who can help relieve general symptoms of tension.

Massage as part of a slimming regime

Therapists specialising in body massage are employed in salons and centres which specialise in weight control programmes. This is not because massage makes clients lose weight, but because they benefit in other ways which are helpful to their particular regime.

A typical client visiting a health or fitness centre will, after a full consultation and possibly a medical check-up, be given advice on an exercise and diet regime aimed at achieving a weight loss of not more than 2 lb, (less than 1 kg) per week.

There are, of course, many treatments offered by beauty salons which aim to improve and help to reshape the figure alongside diet and exercise.

The role of massage in this field is different. Massage can help motivate a client to stick to the diet and exercise regime. It can help clients' self-image and their consciousness of the state of their body. The touch and attention of the therapist makes them more aware of their posture and stance, important factors in looking good. It can also help clients who have a distorted idea of their size as it often is the case that slimmers think themselves plumper than they are.

Massage does not 'break down' fat. The more direct effects are the stimulation of the circulation to the skin and subcutaneous tissues, improving the texture and look of the skin.

A common complaint sometimes, but not always, associated with overweight is localised deposits of fatty tissue which do not easily respond to diet. This condition is known in the beauty business as cellulite, and should not to be confused with cellulitis which is a medical condition of inflammation of the tissues and like all inflammatory conditions is a contraindication to massage.

Cellulite tends to occur mainly in women and appears on the waist, hips, buttocks, thighs, inner knee, upper arm and the upper back. It often looks lumpy and dimples on pressure and will frequently feel colder to the touch than surrounding tissue.

> **REMEMBER**
> Always check with the client as fatty tissue, and particularly cellulite, is often much more sensitive than you might think.

A body massage is adapted for a client who is overweight or who has cellulite by spending more time on the areas worst affected. Stimulating movements such as pounding and hacking should be included to soften hard fatty areas and stimulate local circulation. The effleurage and petrissage movements can be made firmer and brisker to stimulate the lymphatic and general circulatory systems.

Massage to stimulate lymphatic drainage

> **ACTIVITY**
> Make sure you understand the arrangement of the lymphatic vessels and nodes. Check the direction of lymphatic drainage (see figures 4.11 and 4.12 on page 39).

All massage will stimulate the lymphatic drainage to some extent but occasionally a specific part of the body, usually the legs, will benefit from more specific massage aimed to reduce water retention and puffiness.

- Always remove any restrictive clothing.
- If possible elevate the part to be treated for a time (10–30 minutes) before the massage.
- Elevate the limb or part no more than 25 degrees during the massage.
- Always work on the most proximal part first, working down the limb a handbreadth at a time.
- Think of the limb as a four-sided tube to be emptied and work with hands on opposite sides so that first a movement is performed thoroughly with the hands on the top and bottom surfaces of the limb, then on opposite sides.
- Start each movement lightly, slowly getting deeper as the area softens.

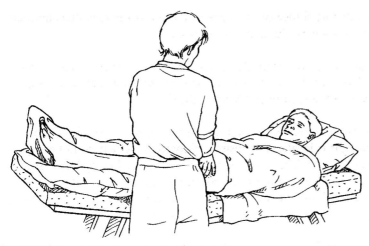

Figure 7.10 *Elevating the legs to assist lymphatic drainage*

- Massage strokes that are appropriate are:
    - a) to soften the area
        - slow, double-handed kneading, compressing the limb gently between the hands;
        - slow gentle picking up;
    - b) to drain the area
        - single-handed vibrations with the other hand giving counter pressure;
        - effleurage towards the nearest lymph nodes.
- On small parts, such as the ankle and foot, thumb kneading and stroking should be used.
- When the limb has been treated section by section, effleurage to the whole limb may be used to end the massage.

SAFE PRACTICE

Massage for a client with the condition known as lymphoedema should not be undertaken without checking that massage is not contraindicated. Lymphoedema is a condition where the lymphatic drainage is no longer effective in draining the limb concerned; it may be a result of lifesaving treatment for cancer which has destroyed lymph nodes or may occur for unknown reasons. The limb affected will be very swollen and hard and care must be taken not to damage the skin which can be vulnerable to infection.

Massage to a limb affected by lymphoedema should only be given by a therapist who is highly trained in manual lymph drainage (MLD) techniques. MLD is usually part of a complex programme of treatment which includes bandaging, exercise and very specialised massage. Deep Swedish-style massage may cause more harm than good.

When massage is applied to a limb affected by lymphoedema it must be gentle and superficial, as deep rough movements may damage the tissues and increase the swelling. The strokes must always be in the direction of lymphatic drainage and towards unaffected areas. If a client with lymphoedema asks for massage, advice should be sought from a lymphoedema clinic before treatment.

Sports massage

There has been a resurgence of interest in massage as an aid to athletes in the last decade. With many more people becoming concerned about health and fitness, they are taking a much more active part in sports, often as very keen amateurs. This increased participation has led to a demand for ways to improve performance and the part-time sportsman today may be as competitive as a professional may have been a few years ago. As training builds up progressively a point can be reached where the body is no longer able to fully recover between sessions and performance will level off or even decline. At this stage, the body is vulnerable to injury if changes in the regime are not made. Massage can be used in reducing muscle tone and tension, reducing muscular discomfort and promoting local and general relaxation, all of which can help prevent injury. Manual massage has a long tradition in many countries, and athletes in the past used to take advantage of this treatment long before physiotherapists and osteopaths existed. Many modern sports men and women have become excellent massage therapists because they have a real understanding of the anatomy and physiology necessary and of the sports concerned.

Uses of massage in sport

- For general treatment to maintain muscles in good condition by increasing the circulation in the muscles.
- Pre-event, to prepare muscles for strenuous work and enhance performance.
- Post-event, to restore muscles after strenuous work and assist recovery.
- To treat local areas which show incomplete recovery from injury.

General treatment

Ideally, a competitive sportsman will have massage at least once a week, preferably after the hardest training session of the week and it should always be followed by one or two days of lighter training. When massage is given once a week it must be deep and thorough, whereas if done more often it can be lighter. Massage should be more frequent at the beginning of the training season than at the end.

Massage should always be tailored to each individual athlete and their particular needs.

As the aim of this massage is relaxation and improvement of the circulation to muscles, the routine can follow the general directions for body massage using the same type of strokes.

- Effleurage and stroking movements can be used especially to feel for tension in particular muscles. Deep stroking movements can be applied to individual muscles along the length of the muscle fibres.
- Petrissage movements should start superficially and increase in depth as superficial muscles relax.
- Tapotement/percussion movements should not be too heavy or sharp just because the muscles look so firm.

Vibrations and shakings are particularly useful in treating tense muscles.

- A vibration movement can be applied using the hand or the fingers depending on the size of the area being treated and when applied with gentle pressure is very relaxing.

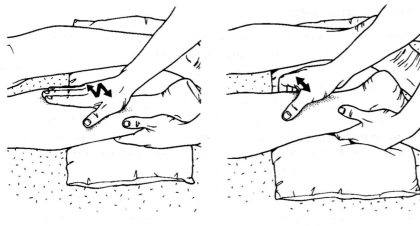

Figure 7.11 *Vibration*   **Figure 7.12** *Shaking*

♦ Shaking movements are applied by using one or both hands to grasp the muscle and shake it from side to side and is useful after deeper movements which may have caused discomfort and tension.

♦ Friction can be used to warm an area before other massage. movements

♦ Frictions applied with the pads of the thumb or fingers, are used on problem areas such as scar tissue or hard bands of muscle which develop as a result of overuse and injury. The frictions will increase local circulation and soften adhesions in the muscle. They should be used only by an experienced sports therapist.

The main adaptations of massage movements when working on sports men and women are to depth and direction. Because of the level of muscle tone and fitness, all movements may be used to a greater depth. Direction is varied according to the effects required. If stimulation of the circulation is needed, then the direction of the strokes will be as usual, but if stretching the muscles is required, then the direction of the muscle fibres must be known and understood.

The hands may be used differently. Whereas in a routine massage the palm of the hand will be in contact for the majority of movements, in a sports massage the thumbs, fingers, heel of the hand and even the elbow may be used to obtain the necessary depth and to concentrate the pressure on a specific area.

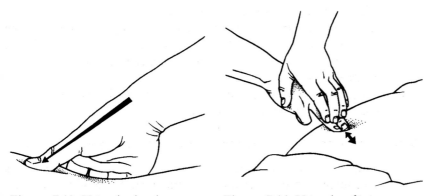

Figure 7.13 *Using the thumb*   **Figure 7.14** *Using deep friction*

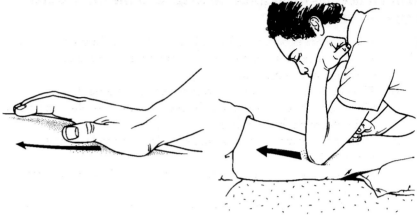

Figure 7.15 *Using the heel of the hand*   **Figure 7.16** *Using the elbow*

Progress Check

Try out all the techniques shown on a client who is fit and has very firm muscles.

Pre-event massage
Only light massage should be given before an event. No deep massage movements should be used for four or five days before a competition or important training session. It has been shown that some heavy massage strokes, especially percussion, produce an immediate decrease in muscle performance and an increase of creatine kinase in the blood suggesting muscle damage.

Post-event massage
The purpose of massage after exercise is to help the removal of the waste products of the activity from the muscles and the sooner this is carried out the better. If the athlete waits too long then the muscles to be worked on may be stiff and sore, making the massage much more uncomfortable. The rate of work should be slow with the depth increasing gradually as superficial muscles relax. Avoid all percussion movements.

To treat local areas which show incomplete recovery from injury
This is usually work undertaken by specialised therapists with a medical background such as osteopaths and chartered physiotherapists, but massage therapists might well find themselves working with such staff to the benefit of both. Acute sporting injuries should never be treated by unqualified personnel.

Muscle stretching is an important part of the athlete's fitness regime and exercises will be devised to stretch individual and groups of muscles. When a muscle is stretched along its length as in exercise, the fibres are drawn closer together. Massage can stretch a muscle in any direction and so can be used to separate bundles of muscle fibres by working across them. Deep frictions applied across the muscle fibres can also be used to soften deep scar tissue which may be present in soft tissue as a result of old injuries.

Differences between sports massage and the more usual types of massage

◆ The massage is being performed on people who know a great deal about their bodies and to whom even a minor degree of malfunction is noticeable.

◆ The bodies being treated are very fit, strong and hard.

◆ Effleurage is used but to a much lesser extent; it is often diagnostic as the therapist feels for problems.

◆ Most movements are on specific muscles or muscle groups, superficial and deep.

◆ Knowledge of the musculo-skeletal structure of the area is very important.

◆ Knowledge of the muscles used in specific sports or activities is an advantage.

Points to be considered in treating athletes

◆ Use a couch which is firm and strong, preferably one where the height can be altered as you will need to exert a greater degree of force than usual.

◆ Posture and stance should enable the therapist to exert pressure where needed – work close to the couch and use your body weight.

◆ To reach deeper muscles, you need to work through superficial muscles and connective tissue. To avoid the superficial muscles tensing up, start gently and instead of working directly on tender spots approach from different angles.

◆ Even though problems may present in one area, they may be caused by or cause problems in another, for example if the problem is in the foot, treat the whole leg and look at the lower back; if in the shoulder, check the neck region.

> **REMEMBER**
> Many disabled people are fine athletes too.

> **ACTIVITY**
> Make a list of five sports that friends participate in. Work out the main muscle groups that are likely to be used most often in these sports and list how you would alter your usual massage routine to treat a person who participates in each.

> **Key Terms**
> You need to know what these words mean. Go back through the chapter or check in the glossary to find out.
>
> ◆ Bonding
> ◆ Cellulite
> ◆ Cellulitis
> ◆ Eye contact
> ◆ Lymphoedema
> ◆ Muscle tone
> ◆ Obesity
> ◆ Pre-event
> ◆ Rheumatism

After working through this chapter you will be able to:

- appreciate how ancient pressure techniques can be integrated into current practice
- describe the basic techniques of shiatsu
- integrate some shiatsu pressures into practical massage
- describe the theoretical basis of reflexology
- integrate some reflex techniques into a foot or hand massage
- recognise the origins of Ayurvedic techniques
- apply some of the techniques used in Indian head massage.

NB Remember that this chapter gives only an introduction to the therapies described.

In the Eastern countries of the world, different forms of massage have always been part of healing and medical practice. This continues in the East today often combined with modern Western methods of treatment.

In China, Japan and India, techniques using pressures on parts of the body have long been used and are now being accepted in the West. Three of these massage methods are particularly appropriate to be absorbed and integrated with orthodox methods of Western massage especially with aromatherapy. These are shiatsu, reflexology and Indian head massage.

Shiatsu

The Japanese word *shiatsu* (*shi*: finger, *atsu*: pressure) describes pressures on the points that are used for acupuncture so that shiatsu-type movements are often called acupressures. Pressure is applied to points using the thumbs, fingers, other parts of the hand and even the elbows or feet.

A shiatsu treatment is very different from the usual Swedish-style massage. No oil is used and there are no smooth flowing strokes, just pressure and stretching. A true shiatsu massage can be given through the clothes with the client lying on a well-carpeted floor. However, some shiatsu-type pressures applied with the fingers, thumb or elbow can be integrated into a Western-style massage very successfully and more can be used as a knowledge of the meridian lines is gained. Sliding pressures applied with the thumb or the hand along meridians are particularly useful when oils are being used.

Shiatsu massage is just one part of a whole philosophy of treatment attempting to return the energy or chi of the body to a state where Yin (negative) and Yang (positive) qualities are in balance. It is based on the theory that a person's chi flows through the body in well-defined paths or channels which are called meridians. There are 14 main meridians each related to and affecting a major organ of the body.

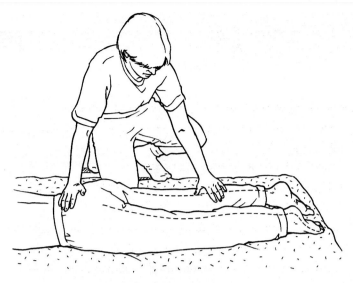

Figure 8.1 *Thumbing the bladder meridian in the leg*

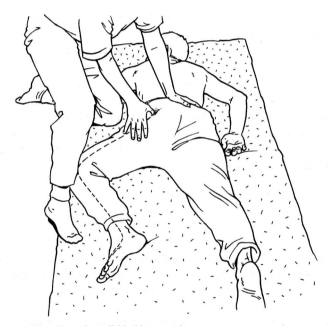

Figure 8.2 *Thumbing the gall bladder meridian*

When in good mental and physical health, energy should flow smoothly through the meridians with the Yin and Yang qualities balanced. Yin qualities are described as dark, cool, moist, soft, receptive and feminine, while Yang characteristics are light, hot, dry, hard, active and masculine. The Yin meridians are on the front of the body with the energy flowing upwards, while the Yang meridians are on the back of the body with the energy flowing downwards.

The meridians link the organs together and seem to interact with each other. If the energy flowing through the meridians is disturbed or interrupted, then the associated organs don't function properly and the

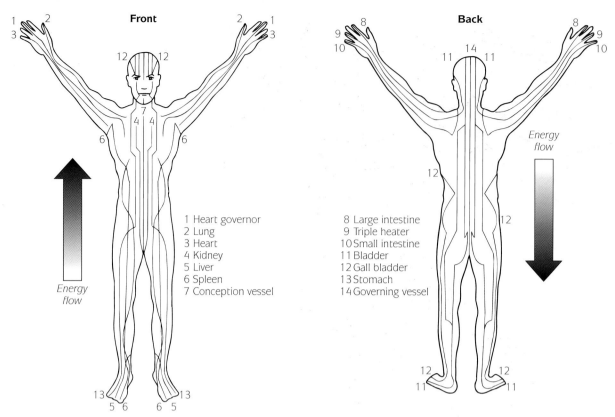

Figure 8.3 *The meridian system*

Front

1 Heart governor
2 Lung
3 Heart
4 Kidney
5 Liver
6 Spleen
7 Conception vessel

8 Large intestine
9 Triple heater
10 Small intestine
11 Bladder
12 Gall bladder
13 Stomach
14 Governing vessel

Back

Energy flow

person may become unwell. Acupoints are situated along the course of the meridians and are said to be the points at which the energy flow along the meridians can be affected, by needling in the case of acupuncture, or pressure in the case of acupressure

Pressures

The thumbs are the usual tools for applying pressures as the acu points are mostly placed in thumb-sized hollows, but in some areas a finger may be used often supported by the adjacent finger. The heel of the hand or elbow may be used over larger areas such as the side of the buttocks.

Pressure should be applied in a firm, controlled manner with body weight controlling the amount of pressure. No poking or roughness should be used and pressure should be moderate to light, building up quite slowly and steadily. When sliding pressure is applied, it should be even and the sliding movement steady, with care being taken not to cause discomfort by pulling on hair or skin.

When pressure is applied to the back or chest, the client should breath out and then breath in when the pressure is released. It is also appropriate to adjust the pressures to the rate of breathing when working on the face.

Pressures are usually performed once only over the area whereas the traditional massage movements will be repeated a number of times depending on the time available and the speed of the strokes.

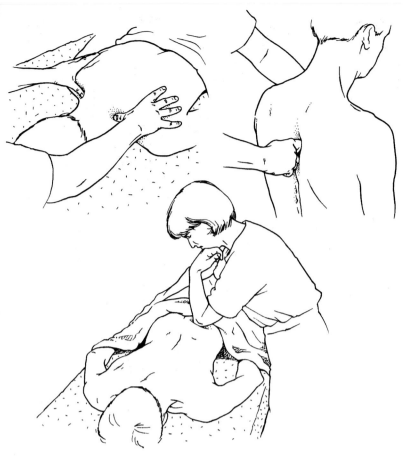

Figure 8.4 *Acupressure stimulation with the thumbs, the knuckle or the elbow*

There are hundreds of acu points in the body, but some are much more commonly stimulated than others. The points are symmetrical on the left and right sides of the body and are named for the meridians that they lie on. When pressure is applied to them, they tend to be more sensitive than the surrounding tissues.

Any of these pressures can be integrated into a massage routine and would be especially useful in an aromatherapy treatment. Care must be taken not to use too much oil to prevent sliding off the acu points.

A full shiatsu treatment carried out by a shiatsu practitioner would include breathing exercises, relaxation techniques, shaking and gentle rocking movements as well as pressures along the meridians at the back and front of the body. Passive movements of the limbs are also used to put major joints through their full range.

For details of professional training courses in shiatsu contact The Shiatsu Society of the UK (see page 252, 'Useful Addresses').

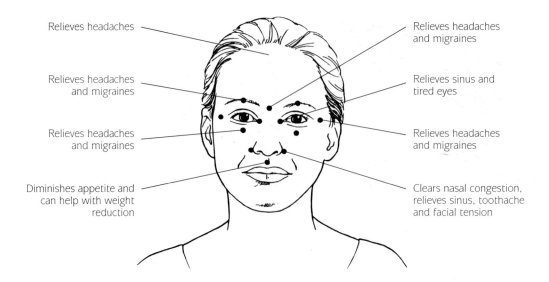

Figure 8.5 *Common acupressure points in the face*

Relieves headaches

Relieves headaches and migraines

Relieves headaches and migraines

Diminishes appetite and can help with weight reduction

Relieves headaches and migraines

Relieves sinus and tired eyes

Relieves headaches and migraines

Clears nasal congestion, relieves sinus, toothache and facial tension

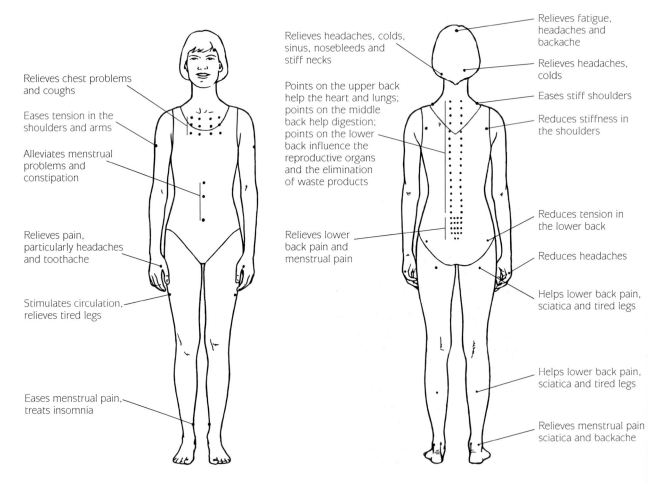

Relieves chest problems and coughs

Eases tension in the shoulders and arms

Alleviates menstrual problems and constipation

Relieves pain, particularly headaches and toothache

Stimulates circulation, relieves tired legs

Eases menstrual pain, treats insomnia

Relieves headaches, colds, sinus, nosebleeds and stiff necks

Points on the upper back help the heart and lungs; points on the middle back help digestion; points on the lower back influence the reproductive organs and the elimination of waste products

Relieves lower back pain and menstrual pain

Relieves fatigue, headaches and backache

Relieves headaches, colds

Eases stiff shoulders

Reduces stiffness in the shoulders

Reduces tension in the lower back

Reduces headaches

Helps lower back pain, sciatica and tired legs

Helps lower back pain, sciatica and tired legs

Relieves menstrual pain sciatica and backache

Figure 8.6 *Some common acupressure points*

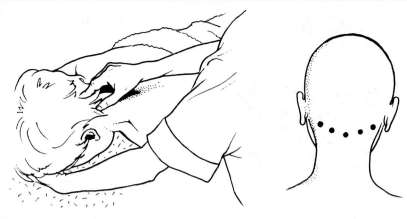

Figure 8.7 *Pressures to base of skull*

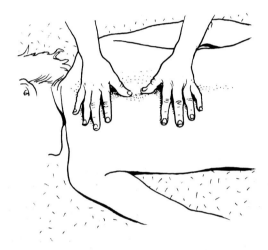

Figure 8.8 *Sliding pressures down side of spine*

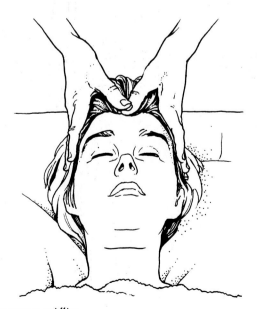

Figure 8.9 *Pressures to midline*

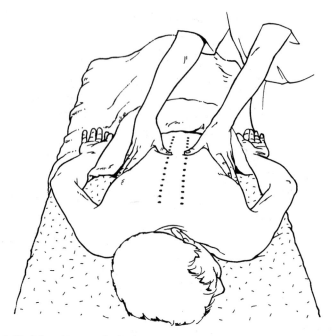

Figure 8.10 *Thumbing on the back*

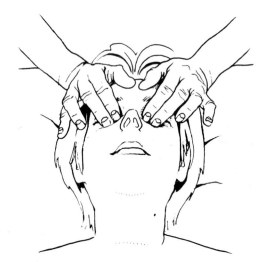

Figure 8.11 *Finger pressures on cheek bones*

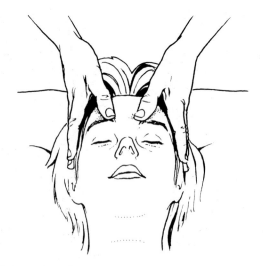

Figure 8.12 *Pressures to eyebrows*

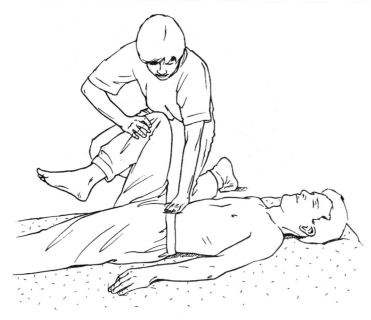

Figure 8.13 *Passive movement, single leg rotation*

Reflexology

Reflexology is not massage in the general sense of the word but is the application of specific pressures to reflex points in the feet and hands, most commonly the feet.

The theory behind the effectiveness of reflexology is very similar to that of shiatsu. According to the principles of both techniques there are energy lines running vertically from head to foot.

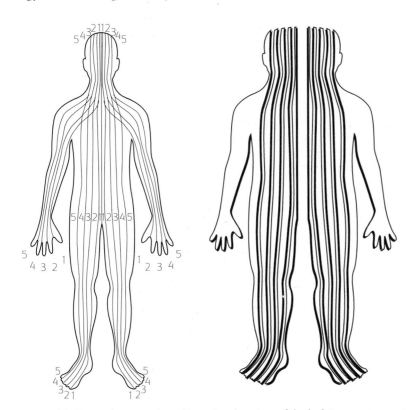

Figure 8.14 *Zones shown as three-dimensional sections of the body*

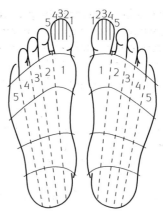

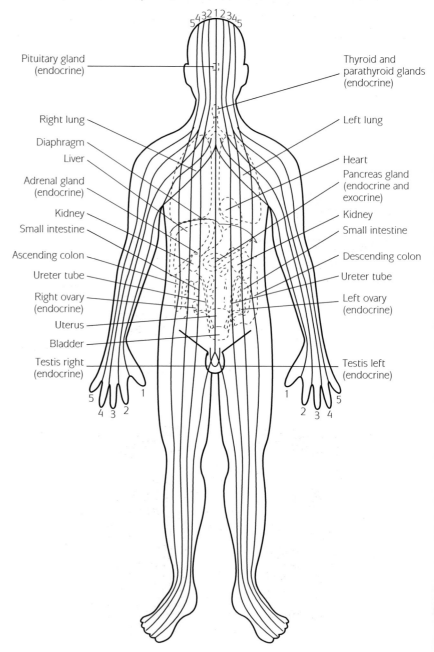

Figure 8.15 *Zone areas on the feet. Note that all five zones are found on the big toe and each small toe repeats and 'magnifies' the zone of the relevant head area*

Pituitary gland (endocrine)

Thyroid and parathyroid glands (endocrine)

Right lung

Left lung

Diaphragm

Liver

Heart

Adrenal gland (endocrine)

Pancreas gland (endocrine and exocrine)

Kidney

Kidney

Small intestine

Small intestine

Ascending colon

Descending colon

Ureter tube

Ureter tube

Right ovary (endocrine)

Left ovary (endocrine)

Uterus

Bladder

Testis right (endocrine)

Testis left (endocrine)

Figure 8.16 *Placement of major organs and glands within the zones*

It is said that the body can be influenced by pressures on points along these lines. In shiatsu, stimulation is applied along the meridian lines all over the body but, in reflexology, only on the soles and dorsum of the feet or hands. The points on the feet and hands are known as reflex points which are believed to relate quite closely to organs and structures of the body.

Although foot massage treatments have been recorded in ancient times, modern reflexology has developed from a system of zone therapy discovered and practised in the USA in the 1920s and 30s.

Zone therapy divided the body into 10 zones or energy channels running vertically through the body from the feet to the head, five on each side, one for each finger or toe. Any organ, gland or body part lying in a certain zone will have its reflex point in the corresponding zone of the foot or hand. This allows a 'map' of the body to be drawn across the soles and other parts of the feet and hands showing the corresponding organs of the body.

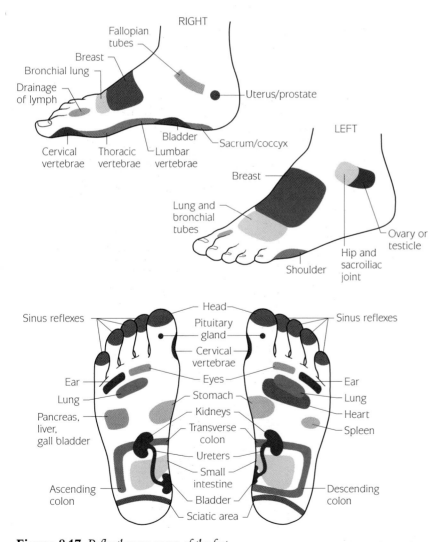

Figure 8.17 *Reflextherapy zones of the feet*

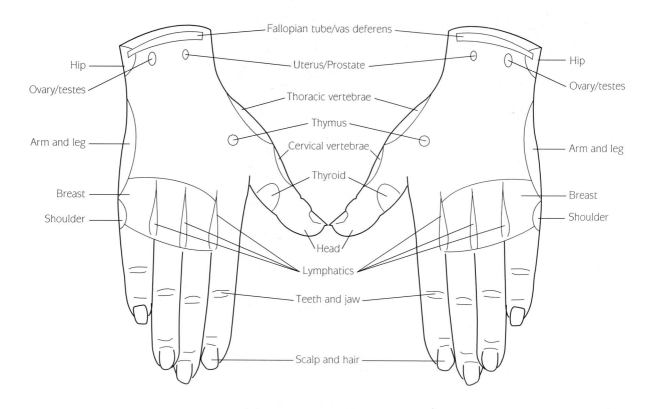

Right hand (dorsal view)
Left hand (dorsal view)

Fallopian tube/vas deferens
Hip
Uterus/Prostate
Hip
Ovary/testes
Thoracic vertebrae
Ovary/testes
Thymus
Arm and leg
Cervical vertebrae
Arm and leg
Thyroid
Breast
Breast
Shoulder
Shoulder
Head
Lymphatics
Teeth and jaw
Scalp and hair

Right hand (palmar view)
Left hand (palmar view)

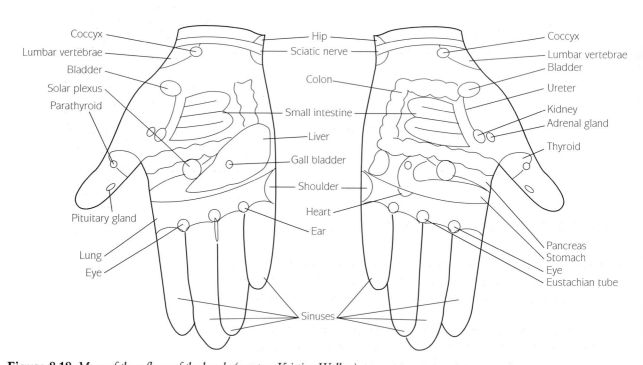

Coccyx
Hip
Coccyx
Lumbar vertebrae
Sciatic nerve
Lumbar vertebrae
Bladder
Bladder
Solar plexus
Colon
Ureter
Parathyroid
Kidney
Small intestine
Adrenal gland
Liver
Thyroid
Gall bladder
Shoulder
Pituitary gland
Heart
Pancreas
Ear
Stomach
Lung
Eye
Eye
Eustachian tube
Sinuses

Figure 8.18 *Maps of the reflexes of the hands (courtesy Kristine Walker)*

A clear example of the relationship of body structures to the foot is shown in the diagram of the spine superimposed on the inner border of the foot (Figure 8.19).

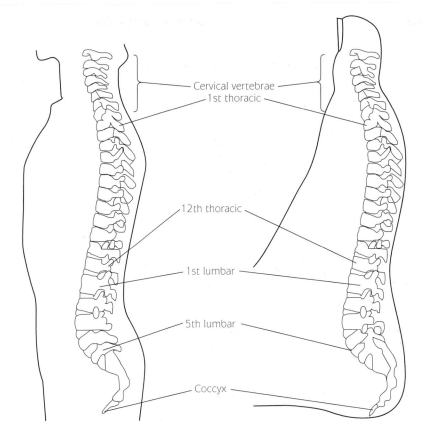

Figure 8.19 *Reflex area for the spine showing relationship of spine reflex to spine in the body*

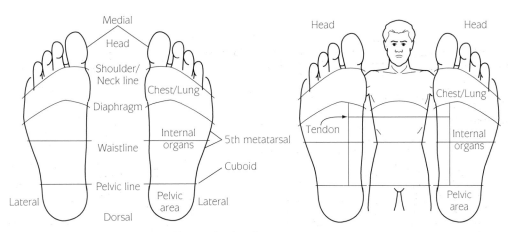

Figure 8.20 *The major areas of the foot divided by the 'landmarks'*

Reflexology techniques can be described as powerful tools for health and healing but they should not be used for diagnosing illnesses or treating them except by fully qualified reflexologists working in a medical setting.

The method of applying pressures in reflexology is very different from shiatsu, the most common method being a rhythmic 'walking' of the thumb (or finger) over the area. This combines a pressure phase with a relaxation phase as the thumb moves forward staying in contact with the skin all the time. The first joint of the thumb is flexed then straightened as it creeps over the area being treated with most of the pressure being applied with the edge of the thumb not the tip. Pressure is applied at an angle of about 45 degrees, not directly, down into the foot tissue.

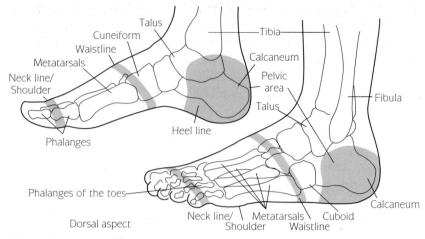

Figure 8.21 *Areas of the foot (shown in grey) superimposed on a diagram of the bones*

(a)   (b)

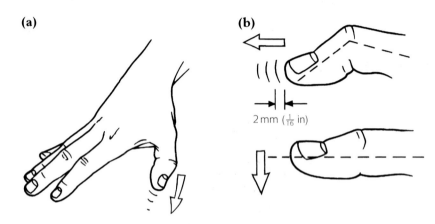

Figure 8.22 *a) Thumb walking technique: flex the thumb at first joint and move forward in very small stages (2 mm/$\frac{1}{16}$in). Practise until you can move incrementally while keeping the shoulders and arm relaxed. b) Thumb walking showing pressure phase – directed down and in – and relax phase*

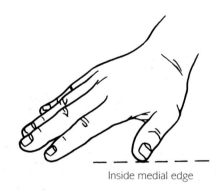

Inside medial edge

Figure 8.23 *Thumb walking practice using inside medial edge*

ACTIVITY

Practise the reflexology technique on yourself. Sit in a chair and practise thumb 'walking' on your thigh. Feel the pressure and relaxation phases and the gentle forward movement of your thumb which seems to happen without any effort to push it forward.

In a reflexology treatment, the foot must be relaxed before the pressures are started. This is often achieved by some general massage strokes such as effleurage to the foot or by passive movements such as ankle rolling or shaking of the foot with a vibration movement.

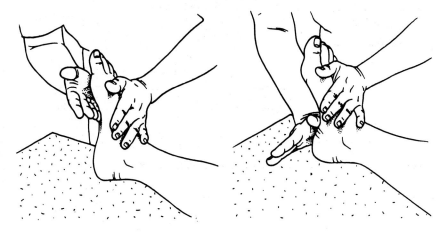

Figure 8.24 *Effleurage to the foot*

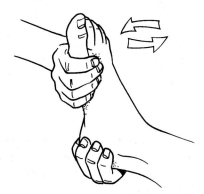

Figure 8.25 *Ankle rotations*

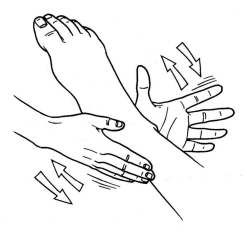

Figure 8.26 *Shimmie vibrations to the ankles*

> **REMEMBER**
> The foot must be fully supported during a treatment and when pressures are applied with one hand, the other must be holding the foot in the optimum position for treatment. This hand may also be used to draw the foot towards or onto the working thumb.

Any other relaxing massage movements, such as thumb stroking or kneading to the sole of the foot, may be useful to aid relaxation.

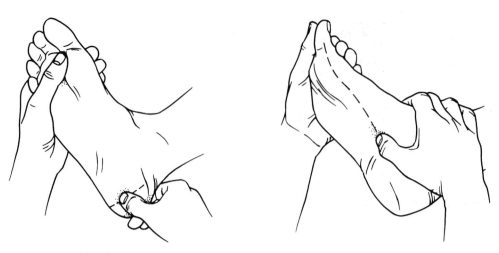

Figure 8.27 *Support holds: left hand supports and positions the foot*

The 'walking' movements can be performed for a general treatment covering all the zones of the foot in sequence or as a treatment for specific problems by concentrating on particular areas of the foot.

A general treatment may follow a set sequence of movements but should be adapted to the client's particular needs.

A possible sequence may be:

◆ a full consultation
◆ the client made comfortable, seated or half lying with the feet facing the therapist
◆ relaxation techniques carried out on both feet.

Treatment is then started on one foot.

◆ Work on the 'chest' area on the plantar and dorsal surfaces of the foot.

(a)   **(b)**

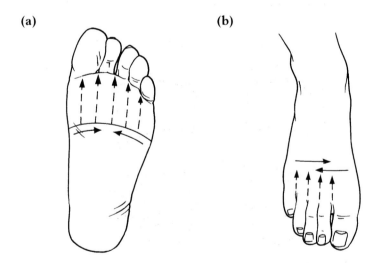

Figure 8.28 *a) Chest area, plantar aspect b) Chest area, dorsal aspect*

◆ Work the head and neck area by moving over the plantar surface of each toe.

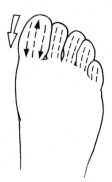

Figure 8.29 *Head and neck areas: work up and down the toes*

● Work the upper 'abdominal' region.

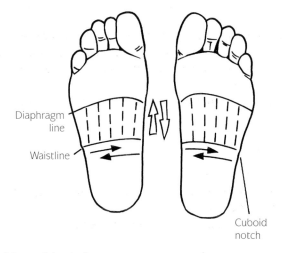

Diaphragm line

Waistline

Cuboid notch

Figure 8.30 *Upper abdominal area*

● Work the lower 'abdominal' region.

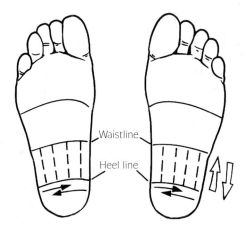

Waistline

Heel line

Figure 8.31 *Lower abdominal area*

● Work along the reflex zone that includes the urinary system.

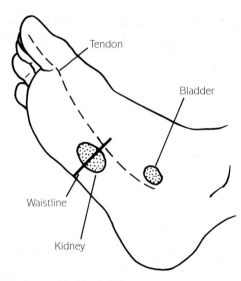

Figure 8.32 *Urinary area, bladder to kidney*

🔹 Work around the ankle to cover the 'reproductive' zone.

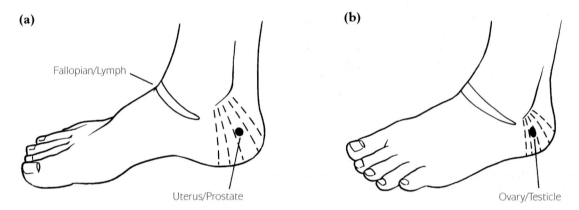

(a)

(b)

Figure 8.33 *a) Lymph and reproductive reflexes, medial view b) Pelvic area and reproductive reflexes, lateral view*

🔹 Work the 'spinal' zone along the inner border of the foot.

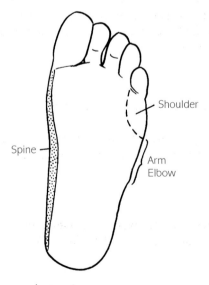

Figure 8.34 *Spine area, plantar view*

- Finish with pressure applied to the 'solar plexus' region of the feet asking the client to breath out as pressure is applied and to breath in as pressure is released.
- Repeat on the other foot.

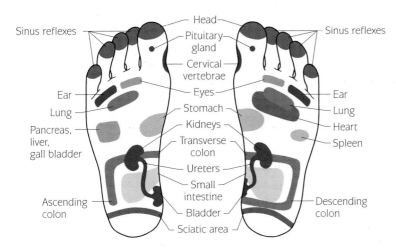

Figure 8.35 *Reflexology zones of soles of the feet*

It is usual for the client to feel tender areas or even soreness or pain in some of the reflex zones. This indicates an imbalance in the energy flow in that zone and sometimes can be related to physical symptoms that the client has noted. A therapist may notice congestion in the form of little grainy or lumpy areas which is also represent imbalance, these may coincide with tender spots and are often referred to as crystals.

If foot treatments are impractical, then hand reflexology may be beneficial with a similar pattern of movements being employed. The pressures used on the hands should be lighter and great care should be taken not to cause pain.

Progress Check

Devise a massage routine for the lower leg and foot that integrates some basic reflex movements into the usual Swedish massage.

For details of professional reflexology courses contact The Association of Reflexologists (see page 252, 'Useful Addresses').

Indian head massage

Indian head massage (IHM) is based on the traditional system of medicine known as Ayurvedic medicine which has been practised in India and Sri Lanka for thousands of years.

Ayurvedic is a Sanskrit word meaning the science of life or knowledge of life, and aims to promote health, natural beauty and long life. It is said to be a complete healing system to balance the mind, body and spirit, and as such it can be said to be truly holistic.

Ayurveda teaches that health is maintained by the balance of energies and in this sense it has much in common with other Eastern healing theories. In the East, the life force has various names: in Japan it is known as *sakia-tundra* or *ki*, in China as *chi* and in India it is called *prana*.

Ayurveda teaches that the five basic elements present in all living creatures are air, fire, water, earth and ether. It teaches that these elements are represented in the body by three energies or *doshas* known as *vata*, *pitta* and *kapha*. These are considered to be the invisible forces that co-ordinate the functions of the body, shaping how one looks, functions, thinks and feels. The balance of the doshas varies from one individual to another. An Ayurvedic practitioner will spend a considerable amount of time searching out the *prakruti* of the person being treated, the prakruti being the unique blend of doshas for each person.

In general terms, the qualities of the three types tend to show the following characteristics.

	Vata	Pitta	Kapha
Skin and hair	Dry	Oily	Oily
Skin	Cold	Hot	Hot
Build	Light	Light	Heavy
Mood	Fluctuates	Intense	Stable
Temperament	Creative	Efficient and ambitious	Patient and caring

Table 8.1 *Some characteristics of the three doshas*

As the Ayurvedic system treats the whole person, it includes dietary advice, massage and other treatments tailored specifically for the doshas of each person.

ACTIVITY

If you have friends with an Indian background, ask whether they are familiar with the Ayurvedic philosophy and if massage plays a part in their family routine.

Massage has always been part of everyday life in India. Both men and women often receive a weekly massage as a matter of course. Children are massaged from birth by their mothers which helps the bonding process and the creation of a loving atmosphere in the home. In particular, children and adults benefit from massage to the head and face.

In Indian massage, oils are almost always used which makes their techniques fit in particularly well with a Western aromatherapy treatment.

The oils used for head massage are meant to improve the condition of the hair and scalp and to improve the working of the mind. Sometimes ghee, which is clarified butter, is used, but more often warmed, organic vegetable oils are used. The oils will often be mixed with herbs, spices or fruit extracts and the particular blends will be selected to treat the dominant dosha of a person. This might mean that a vata-type person will be massaged using a 'warming' oil such as mustard and a kapha-type person a 'cooling' oil such as sunflower, each being mixed with herbal extracts. The oil may be left on the scalp for 24 hours to help condition the hair or it may be shampooed off.

Indian head massage is particularly beneficial in balancing the chakras which are said to be the energy centres of the body. There are seven main chakras situated at different levels, running from the 'master' chakra at the crown of the head to the lowest at the base of the spine. Working on these chakras releases tension and restores the balance of energy allowing the body and mind to feel relaxed and rested. Pressures on points over the chakras correspond in many ways to pressures used in shiatsu or acupressure points.

Contraindications
to Indian head massage

- Epilepsy.
- Scalp infections.
- Severe migraine.
- Recent injury to the head or neck (for example a whiplash injury).

Oils for Indian head massage
The oils will always be of organic vegetable origin and are often mixed with essential oils as used in Western aromatherapy techniques. (See chapter 10 for charts of carrier oils.) Oils are selected and mixed to suit the hair and skin of each client. For example, for someone with dry, thin hair and skin – a vata type – it would be appropriate to use an oil such as sweet almond or jojoba mixed with a little avocado and evening primrose oil. If required, essential oils may then be added to suit the client's needs as established after a full aromatherapy consultation. The oil is usually gently warmed for head and face massage.

Although, traditionally, oils are used for Indian head massage, the techniques can be used without, which is often more acceptable to clients in the West.

It is usual to treat the client in the lying position especially when it is part of a more general massage, but many of the movements and pressures can be applied with the client sitting and fully dressed. This is particularly useful in an office or similar environment when a few minutes of massage can improve relaxation and posture leading to a more efficient workforce.

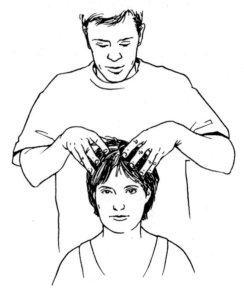

Figure 8.36 *Client sitting*

To start a head, neck and face massage, the therapist stands at the head of the couch. The client should be lying in a comfortable position with a folded towel under the head and perhaps a pillow under the knees to help relaxation.

The first few movements can be carried out without oil.

● Place the hands on the shoulders and wait for the client to relax and for the therapist to feel calm and relaxed.
● 'Open' the chest and shoulders by pressing down on the front of the shoulders asking the client to breathe in as you press and out as you release. This can be done a few times.

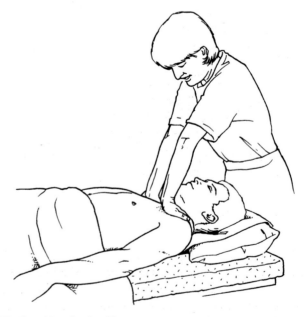

Figure 8.37 *Stretching the shoulders*

- With the palms of the hands press gently over the sternum and circle a few times to comfort the area.
- Take the client's head in both hands and when you are sure that the neck is relaxed, gently rotate the head in one direction then the other
- Support the head with one hand, place the other on top of the shoulder and stretch the neck to the side. Change hands and repeat on the opposite side.

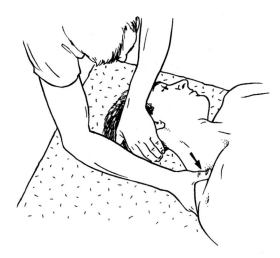

Figure 8.38 *Using one hand to support the head, apply stretch to the trapezius muscle*

- Now apply warm oil to the hands and run the fingers through the hair from the roots to the ends, covering the whole head.
- With the tips of the fingers, apply friction all over the scalp. Start with the fingers at the hairline, move them in deep circular movements so that the scalp moves over the bone. Gradually work backwards until the whole head has been covered.

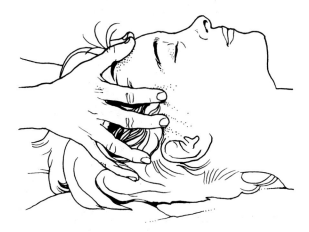

Figure 8.39 *Friction to the scalp*

- One of the main techniques of IHM is pressures with the whole hand to the head. Cup your hands around the head with one hand on the forehead and the other on the crown of the head. Apply pressures with fingertips and palms, moulding the hands to the shape of the head. Press gently at first, squeezing the head so that the pressure is felt gradually. Move the hands around the head applying pressure in different directions.

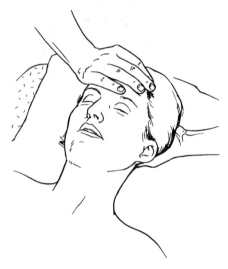

Figure 8.40 *Applying pressure with both hands*

- Grip the sides of the head with the fingers so that the thumbs are at the midline of the hairline. With one thumb resting on the other, apply pressure then release. Repeat, moving backwards over the crown of the head to the base of the occipital bone.

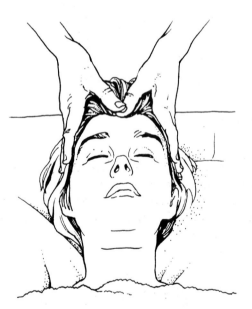

Figure 8.41 *Pressure to midline*

- Repeat the above with the thumbs a half inch to the sides of the centre moving from hairline to occipital bone.
- Rest the thumbs midway and slightly above the eyebrows. Rest the palms around both sides of the head. Hold for a short time and release.
- Rest the fingers on the temples with thumbs together between the eyebrows. Apply pressures along the length of the eyebrows then repeat an inch higher until the whole forehead is covered.

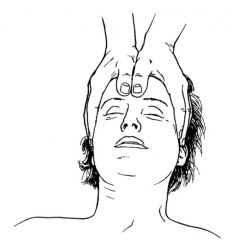

Figure 8.42 *Hold and release*

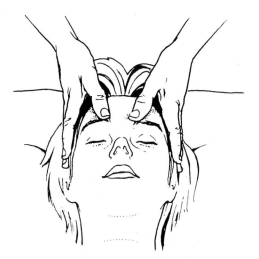

Figure 8.43 *Pressures to eyebrows*

♦ With the middle fingers over the mastoid process behind the ear
(known as the karna point) gently massage with circular
movements over the process. Then, using the right hand, progress
along the base of the skull to the midline. Change hands and
repeat on the left side.

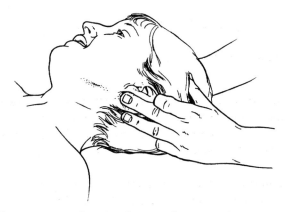

Figure 8.44 *Massage over the mastoid process (karna point)*

- With the fingertips as if playing the piano, cover the underside of the lower jaw and the neck with small tapping movements.
- Repeat the first and second movements, running fingers through the length of the hair and applying friction to the scalp.
- End the treatment with the hands resting over the closed eyes. Leave the hands for a few moments then lift gently away.

SAFE PRACTICE

Take care that essential oils are not applied to the eyelids and do not get in the eyes.

Progress Check

Integrate just a few of these movements into your usual facial or neck and chest massage routine.

There are many more pressures and other techniques related to specific points on the face and head. Many of them can be integrated into a full Western-style massage to great effect.

Key Terms

You need to know what these words mean. Go back through the chapter or check in the glossary to find out.

- acupressure
- Ayurvedic
- chi
- dosha
- meridian
- prakruti
- prana
- reflex point
- Yang
- Yin
- zones

AROMATHERAPY

9

After working through this chapter you will be able to:

- define aromatherapy
- recognise the historical role of plants and plant-based healing
- describe the development of aromatherapy as a complementary therapy
- list characteristics shared by complementary therapies
- describe the factors which may affect the absorption of essential oils through the skin
- explain the relationship between the sense of smell and memory
- list the aims of the consultation process
- develop a consultation technique specific to aromatherapy
- recognise the contraindications to aromatherapy treatment.

Aromatherapy is the name given to holistic treatments that use essential oils of plants for healing and to improve physical and emotional well-being.

Plants have always been used by man for medicinal purposes from the distant past to the present time. Most parts of the world will have a history of using their indigenous plants for medicinal and cosmetic purposes. In the Middle East and Far East, exotic-sounding plants such as myrrh and frankincense were grown and used and are recorded in the Bible and other writings. Indian literature from 2000 BC lists hundreds of plant substances such as cinnamon, ginger, myrrh, coriander and sandalwood, many of which are still used in Ayurvedic medicine today.

Aromatic materials were used in many parts of the world for thousands of years for purposes other than medicinal such as embalming the dead. We can see proof of that today in the archaeological finds of containers and in ancient paintings and writings. The Egyptians set great store by the use of perfumed substances for ceremonial and everyday use. Traces of the contents of ointment and cosmetic jars have been found in excavations of the Pyramids.

The use of aromatic substances is recorded in Babylon where gardens of medicinal plants were planted as a source of materials for treating disease. This knowledge of the uses of aromatics spread from Egypt throughout the Mediterranean with the Greeks acquiring much of their medicinal knowledge from the Egyptians. The Greeks then developed many of their own methods using local herbs, fruits and flowers.

Hippocrates lists huge numbers of plants in use for medicinal purposes.

Many Greek doctors lived and worked in Rome, Galen being one of them. Essential oils of plants were used there for many purposes. Wealthy Romans used aromatics to perfume their hair and bodies and scented oils were used for massage after bathing.

The Chinese also have an ancient herbal tradition which was used alongside the practice of acupuncture. The burning of aromatics was part of religious ceremonies as it is still in many parts of the world today and in many religions of the world.

The Arabs are believed to have developed distillation as a method of extracting oils from plants towards the end of the first millennium and the perfumes of Arabia became famous throughout Europe. In Europe, flourishing distillation and perfumery businesses grew up in centres such as Grasse in France which were situated close to the source of plants valued for their aromas and other qualities.

In Southern Africa, many plants, some of which we know as house plants are still used as healing remedies. The English names of some of them will be familiar: mother-in-law's tongue and bitter aloe, for instance. Other indigenous herbs such as wild garlic, wild sage, sour fig and many more are still used today and can be seen growing in the Kirstenbosch gardens in Capetown with their labels showing traditional usages.

Many towns and cities today have botanical gardens showing how local plants were used before the development of modern medicines. In Australia, pride of place goes to plants in the tea tree (*Melaleuca*) family and the many varieties of eucalyptus.

In Europe too, many wild plants were known to local men and women and used to heal wounds and help restore health. In England, the famous botanist Nicholas Culpeper, who practised medicine in the 17th century, published his *Herbal* listing over 300 medicines obtained from English herbs. Around this time, plants were collected and grown in special gardens for use in the expanding cities and collections can still be seen today in botanical gardens such as the Chelsea Physic Garden and Kew Gardens in London where there are extensive collections of plants carefully labelled with their ancient uses.

By the start of the 20th century many more modern drugs were being discovered and developed which reduced the role of plant-based medicine. However, many of today's drugs originate from plant material either directly or through synthetic equivalents, the most famous being aspirin (originally derived from the willow) and digitalis (originally derived from the foxglove). There is growing interest in medical circles in finding new plants which can be exploited for medicines or even genetically altered to produce useful new ingredients.

ACTIVITY

If you are interested, try to visit gardens which label medicinal plants and see if any of them are familiar to you as aromatherapy oils or cooking herbs.

The essential oils of plants, obtained by distillation were used in Europe for perfumery, especially in France, and it was a French chemist, Rene-Maurice Gattefosse, who is credited with coining the word aromatherapy in 1928. He became interested in the therapeutic qualities of the oils which appeared to give better results in some cases than their synthetic equivalents. The use of oils was continued by Dr Jean Valnet who found them particularly useful in healing wounds in the Second World War.

Aromatherapy was introduced to Britain in the 1950s by a Madame Arcier through beauty therapy clinics and is still used to a great extent by beauty therapists. Gradually, the therapeutic value of good quality essential oils was recognised and aromatherapy became an important part of complementary therapy. The interest in all complementary therapies continues to grow and aromatherapy is one of the most accessible and user-friendly therapies of them all.

In recent years, the regulation of complementary therapies has become an important issue and in 1991 the Aromatherapy Organisations Council (AOC) was established to act as an umbrella organisation for the professional associations involved in aromatherapy. Currently 12 associations are members of the AOC, some of the largest being:

- Guild of Complementary Practitioners (GCP)
- International Federation of Aromatherapists (IFA)
- International Society of Professional Aromatherapists (ISPA)
- Register of Qualified Aromatherapists (RQA).

These associations have accredited training establishments that teach to the standards set by the AOC. Therapists who complete training in any of these schools may apply to be placed on registers kept by the associations and on one kept by the AOC. They can then be regarded as fully qualified aromatherapists.

ACTIVITY

Look up the AOC website (see page 252, 'Useful Addresses') and gather information of use to an aromatherapist starting to practise.

Aromatherapy is one of the many types of complementary therapies which are becoming much more commonly used both inside and outside the conventional medical care system. Aromatherapy is also widely practised by beauty therapists who are also aromatherapists.

Complementary therapies share a number of characteristics. They:

- help the body to heal itself naturally
- are holistic, that is, they consider the whole person – their physical, emotional and social aspects – when seeking out the causes of problems
- are gentle and having a low risk of side-effects
- give time and opportunity for the patient to develop a relationship through talk and touch
- include the patient in the decision-making process of the treatment.

Aromatherapy satisfies all of these criteria and is often used in conjunction with other therapies such as reflexology, shiatsu or acupressure or some of the Ayurvedic techniques such as Indian head massage.

The benefits of aromatherapy stem from the use of plant products which are most often applied to the body in very small amounts. The products are most commonly the essential oils of plants which are diluted with pure plant oils before being applied to the skin by means of massage. Until the middle of the 20th century, the skin was thought to be fairly impermeable but it is now known that the skin is a poor barrier to lipophilic substances such as the essential oils of plants. Once they have penetrated the skin, the molecules of the essential oils will enter the circulation and lymphatic system and circulate around the body. Many factors determine how much of a chemical penetrates the skin:

- the size of the area of skin to which the oil is applied
- the thickness and permeability of the epidermis in different parts of the body – the epidermis is very thin on the eyelids and parts of the face and is thicker on the legs and trunk
- the number of sweat glands and follicles which allow easy access for the molecules
- damaged skin, as broken or diseased skin will offer no barrier
- warmth – a warm room, warm hands or oil – speeds up absorption, but a body which is too warm and sweating, for example after a sauna, will tend to throw off the oil.

As well as entering the body through the skin, the volatility of essential oils ensures that odour molecules and the aroma will affect the client immediately by entering the nose. The olfactory nerves carry messages from receptor cells in the upper part of the nose to the olfactory bulb which is in direct contact with the limbic system of the brain. The limbic system is a complex inner area of the brain known to be closely linked with emotions and psychological feelings and is instantly affected by smells. It also controls the autonomic nervous system and some hormones.

The part of the limbic system known as the hippocampus is particularly associated with memory, especially in the conversion of short-term memory into long-term memory.

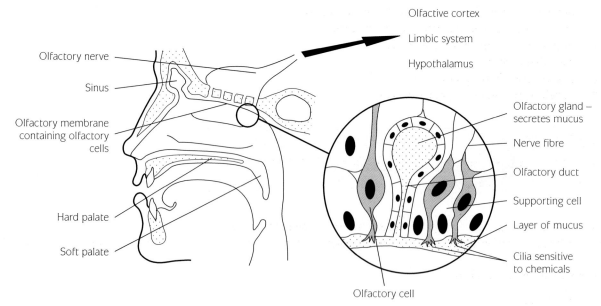

Figure 9.1 *The sense of smell (olfaction)*

One of the most important factors in considering the effects of odours is that of memory. Odours can stimulate memory, enabling people to recall details about events and emotions and very often link them together. This is important in the practice of aromatherapy as an oil which evokes negative or unpleasant memories will be of no benefit while an aroma that evokes pleasant relaxing situations may be of considerable help to the treatment. Everyone reacts to scents differently and the therapist must take this into account during the consultation process.

ACTIVITY

Ask a group of friends which perfumes they like/hate and ask if any smells remind them of anyone or any occasion.

Progress Check

Refer to chapter 4 and re-read the section on skin and the sense of smell.

When you have done this, answer the following questions.

1   What is the relevance of Meissner's corpuscles to massage?
2   Where are the blood vessels located in the skin?
3   What is an allergic response?
4   What is photosensitivity?
5   Where in the brain are smells registered?

Consultation

The consultation process is especially important to clients attending for aromatherapy treatment because the effects of massage and the effects of the essential oils must be considered.

The aims of the consultation are to:

- find out what the client expects from the treatment
- determine what the client needs from the treatment
- ensure that the client is suitable for treatment
- determine any need for special care
- establish rapport
- answer any client queries
- develop and agree a treatment plan.

ACTIVITY

Re-read chapter 3 on consultation procedures for massage treatment.

Information to be gained during the consultation can be summarised under the following headings (see Figure 3.1, page 17, chapter 3).

1 Personal information

- Surname.
- Forenames.

- Address.
- Home telephone number.
- Work telephone number.
- Date of birth.
- Occupation.
- Date of first consultation.

2 Medical details

- Name of doctor.
- Doctor's telephone number.
- General state of health.
- Current medication.
- Current medical treatment.
- Current alternative/complementary treatments.
- Past medical/surgical history with approximate dates.
- General state of health at the time of the consultation.

GOOD PRACTICE

The client should be asked to sign the consultation card to confirm that the information given on personal and medical matters is correct.

REMEMBER

Clients need time to consider the questions. Try not to just tick off a list of possible illnesses. Phrase questions in a variety of ways. A question such as, 'What was the reason for your last visit to the doctor?' might elicit more information.

3 Lifestyle and personality

This gives an overall picture of the person and how they might be helped with an aromatherapy treatment. Questions should not be too direct or probing and whenever possible 'open questions' should be used. The following are examples of open questions.

- What do you feel the problem is?
- How do you think aromatherapy can help you?
- What makes you feel good/bad?

Most questions beginning with 'How', 'Why', 'What', 'Where', 'When' are open questions that will give the client an opportunity to talk. Any question that can be answered by 'Yes' or 'No' is a closed question. Listen to what the client wants and how they perceive their problem.

4 Temperament and emotional state

This is the most challenging part of a consultation and one which will be ongoing throughout treatment. Direct questioning must be tactful and lead the client to discuss problems without feeling that their privacy is being invaded in any way.

REMEMBER

Consultation is ongoing and should be continued throughout the treatment. Information is also gained by observing physical problems and tensions during massage.

One useful way of asking how a client feels emotionally is to ask them to consider how they feel on a scale of 1 to 10 on a bad day, a good day and at the present time.

Any counselling skills that you can acquire will be of real use here in dealing with clients who have problems. Listening skills are of major importance.

Consultation should include a brief explanation of the nature of aromatherapy if the client has not been for treatment before.

Assessment of a client is based on:

- asking appropriate questions and listening carefully and actively to the client's comments
- observation and touch
- experience and intuition.

The information gathered should:

- give you an overall picture of the client
- give you a feel for how you should deal with the client
- direct you to the way in which you can help with problems
- show you how the client can help themselves.

> **ACTIVITY**
>
> Develop a consultation card of your own and use it with colleagues. Ask them to comment constructively on the questions and on your questioning technique and listening skills. You could do the same to help them to develop their consultation process.

Contraindications and precautions

When considering any aromatherapy treatment using massage, then the contraindications and elements of special care related to massage apply:

- when the client is feverish, has an acute infectious disease or is generally unwell
- during the active phase of rheumatoid arthritis
- when the client is being treated for cancer, unless the massage is carried out under medical supervision
- when the client is under the influence of drink or drugs
- if the client is pregnant and you have reason to believe that the pregnancy is unstable.

> **Contraindications**
>
> to localised massage
>
> - Over a limb where there is a history of thrombosis or phlebitis in the blood vessels.
> - Over an area of a skin disorder which may be spread.
> - Over an area of inflammation such as a rash or boil.
> - Over an area of sunburn.
> - Over bruising, cuts, recent scars or abrasions or over very thin, fragile skin.
> - Over recent sprains, fractures or surgical procedures.
> - Over a joint that is hot or swollen.
> - Over any area of swelling.
> - Over very tender or painful muscles.
> - Directly over severe varicose veins.
> - Directly over moles and warts.
> - Over the abdomen during early (first three months) of pregnancy. (Very gentle stroking movements may be used in later stages.)

Conditions where special care should be exercised
Diabetes
In some diabetics circulation is poor, skin sensation may be altered and the skin can become very fragile. The healing process can be very slow, especially in the lower leg and foot.

Epilepsy
Most people with epilepsy have their condition well controlled with medication but especial care must be taken not to leave them unattended on a couch.

Heart disease or blood pressure disorders
Very often a client with these conditions will benefit from massage but the client may need special care. Someone with high blood pressure or heart disease may need to avoid lying flat whereas someone with low blood pressure may feel faint on sitting up and require support. Patients with heart problems should not be massaged over the front of the chest or neck.

Contraindications specific to aromatherapy are usually related to essential oils in general and to the contraindications and precautions of specific oils.

- No essential oils should be taken by mouth
- Essential oils should not be used in the first three months of pregnancy.
- Use of some essential oils may affect medication or homeopathic remedies.
- Citrus oils will cause photosensitivity if they contain furocoumarins.
- Some oils may cause sensitisation or irritation.
- Always check contraindications for individual oils.

Key Terms
You need to know what these words mean. Go back through the chapter or check in the glossary to find out.

- AOC
- Aromatic
- Consultation
- Holistic
- Lipophilic
- Listening skills
- Rapport

ESSENTIAL OILS FOR AROMATHERAPY

After working through this chapter you will be able to:

- define an essential oil
- describe the source of essential oils
- explain the main methods of oil extraction
- outline the factors governing the quality of essential oils
- describe safe methods of storage and preferred labelling of essential oils
- describe the effects of the main chemical categories of essential oils
- describe the main qualities of a selected number of essential oils
- explain the term 'chemotype' and give examples.

As aromatherapy is the name given to treatments that use essential oils once they have been extracted from the plant, it is important for therapists to understand the nature of the oils used. The effects of the oils on the body and mind can be very potent. Oils can be studied to many levels so that some people will call themselves aromatherapists who have only a limited knowledge of essential oils and others will have studied and practised for many years. As more people become aware of the benefits of aromatherapy, training standards are being raised and the levels standardised. As with all complementary therapies, learning is a continuous and continuing process in aromatherapy and should never stop.

ACTIVITY

Re-read chapter 4, with particular reference to aromatherapy, noting references in the sections on the permeability of the skin, sensitisation and allergy and on the nervous system and olfactory receptors.

Because essential oils are said to be good for physical and mental conditions there is a temptation for the practitioner to regard aromatherapy as a form of medicine, but essential oils should not be used as an alternative to prescription medicines. Their particular value is to help maintain people in good health and to improve their well-being and can be especially of use where there are stress-related symptoms or conditions. During consultation, clients should be asked about medical conditions and, if there are any problems, they should always be referred to their doctor.

ACTIVITY

Check your consultation card to make sure there are appropriate medical questions on it.

Essential oils

These are aromatic substances present at very low concentrations in different parts of plants: leaves, flower petals, berries and even twigs. When they are extracted from plants and bottled as pure essential oils, the concentration is 100%. They are available for purchase in this form by the general public as well as aromatherapists and should always be adequately diluted for safe use.

Essential oils are odorous and highly volatile, readily evaporating in the open air. They are quite different from fatty oils, having a constituency more like water than oil. Their chemistry is complex, but they generally contain alcohols, esters, ketones, aldehydes and terpenes. The odiferous materials are formed in the chloroplasts in the leaf and there combine with glucose to form glucosides which are then transported around the plant structures.

The oils are present in tiny droplets in a large number of plants especially those used for their culinary or medicinal properties. Most, but not all, essential oil-bearing plants, such as those in Table 10.1, produce oil only in one part of the plant.

Plant	Part of plant producing oil
Vetiver	Rootlets
Ginger	Rhizome (underground stem)
Sandalwood	Heartwood of tree trunk
Cinnamon	Inner bark of tree
Petitgrain	Twigs and leaves
Ylang ylang	Flowers
Juniper	Whole fruits
Bergamot	Outer rind of fruit (zest)
Fennel	Seeds
Rosemary	Leaves

Table 10.1 *Some plants produce oil in one part of the plant*

Some plants produce different oils in different parts of the same plant for example the plant *Citrus aurantium* var. *amara* is the source for the following oils.

Essential oil	Part of plant
Petitgrain	Leaves and twigs
Bitter orange	Peel
Neroli	Flowers

Table 10.2 Citrus aurantium *var.* amara *is the source of three oils*

The presence of essential oils in orange peel can be demonstrated by squeezing the rind of the fruit next to a lighted match. The oil droplets will spray out and briefly ignite as they pass through the flame. The scent of flowers and herbs is due to their essential oils as is the spiciness of spices.

While they are in the plant, the essences are constantly changing their chemical composition and move from one part of the plant to another according to the time of day and the seasons. This means that the time of harvesting is crucial to the quality of the oils. Other factors which alter the quality of oils in the plants are the soil conditions, variations in climate and methods of cultivation.

Oils used for therapeutic purposes should be grown under strictly organic conditions to avoid contamination with chemicals such as pesticides.

Extraction
Oils are extracted from plants by different methods.

Expression
A few essential oils can be obtained by simple pressure such as the citrus oils – lemon, bergamot, grapefruit and orange – where the oil is contained in the outer part of the skin.

Distillation
The plant parts are heated in water or steam and the vapour given off is cooled to produce a liquid which is a mixture of essential oil and water. The essential oil can easily be separated and drawn off to leave perfumed water behind as a by-product.

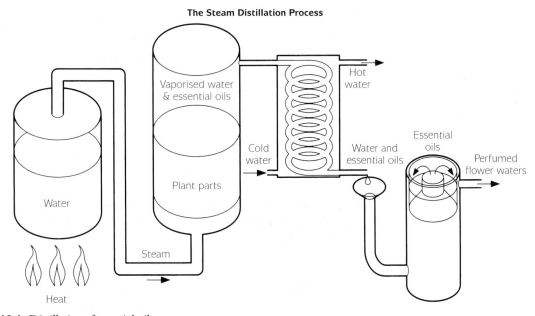

The Steam Distillation Process

Figure 10.1 *Distillation of essential oils*

Solvent extraction
This method is used for some floral oils. The plants are immersed in hydrocarbon solvents to dissolve the essential oils. The solution is then distilled to leave behind a mixture of wax and oil known as a 'concrete'. The wax can then be dissolved by alcohol which in turn can be evaporated off leaving an 'absolute'. Absolutes differ from true essential

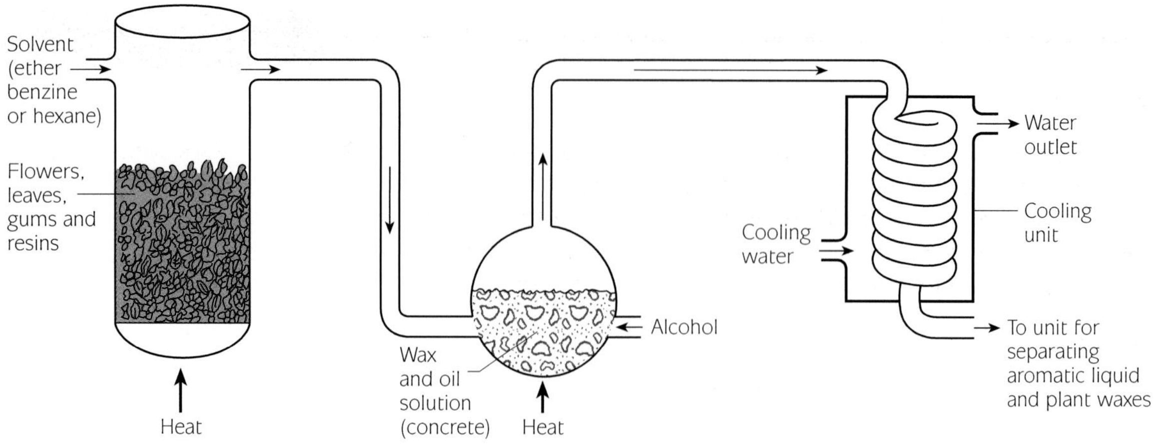
Solvent
(ether
benzine
or hexane)
Flowers,
leaves,
gums and
resins
Heat
Wax
and oil
solution
(concrete)
Heat
Alcohol
Cooling
water
Water
outlet
Cooling
unit
To unit for
separating
aromatic liquid
and plant waxes

Figure 10.2 *Solvent extraction*

oils in that they are generally thicker and more viscous. They are more often used in perfumery than in aromatherapy.

More recently, carbon dioxide has been used as a solvent to extract essential oils successfully. By using carbon dioxide in a state known as hypercritical at high pressure, it becomes a very effective solvent which does not contaminate the oils. This method requires bulky and expensive equipment but the number of essential oils extracted by this method that are commercially available is increasing.

Enfleurage

This traditional method of extraction is used today only for some very expensive oils such as rose and jasmine. It involves spreading the petals of the plant on fat or oil which absorbs the essence and then extracting it from the fat by using solvents to separate them. Even rose and jasmine these days are mostly extracted by the more commercial solvent or distillation methods.

Quality

The quality of essential oils is most important, and care must be taken to use only oils which are pure and unadulterated. The best advice when starting is to deal only with a reputable supplier who is known to stock oils of the highest quality. Good suppliers are also the best source of advice on which oils to order, for example there are a number of different oils called lavender, each with its own qualities.

All plants have a common English name and a recognised botanical Latin name which identifies it more accurately and it is wise to become familiar with the Latin name to avoid mistakes when ordering and using the oils.

Factors which can affect the quality of oils include:

- choice of the best possible member of the plant species
- where the plant was grown
- whether it was grown organically
- how it was harvested and at what time of day
- what method of extraction was used
- how the oils have been stored.

Storage

- Essential oils should be kept in a cool place, at approximately 18°C (65°F). Oils with a high level of terpenes should be kept refrigerated.
- The bottles used should be of dark glass to protect the oil from the light.
- The bottles should not be open-topped but have some form of drop dispenser in the neck.
- All oils should be kept out of the reach of children.

Labelling

All essential oils should be adequately labelled and show the following.

- The full botanical name as well as the common name.
- Instructions for use.
- The quantity of oil in the bottle.
- The name of the company supplying the oil.
- An expiry date.
- Any warnings specific to the oil.
- General warnings, such as 'Not to be taken internally' and 'Keep out of the reach of children'.

Sources of essential oils

All essential oils are obtained from plants. Aromatherapists should gain a knowledge of the plants concerned in order to use the oils to their best effect.

Plants are classified according to principles laid down by Linnaeus in the 18th century. Each plant belongs to a family and is given a generic name (written in italics with a capital initial) and a specific name (lower case italics); for example the full classification of the lavender most commonly used in aromatherapy is shown in Table 10.3.

Kingdom	Plantae
Division	Tracheophyta
Subdivision	Spermatophytina
Class	Angiospermae
Order	Lamiales
Family	Lamiaceae (or Labiatae)
Genus	*Lavandula*
Species	*angustifolia*

Table 10.3 *Botanical classification of common lavender (*Lavandula angustifolia*)*

It is important to identify a plant correctly as there may be others in the genus that are more suitable for medicinal rather than aromatherapy purposes. *Lavandula angustifolia* (see Table 10.3), known as common lavender, is widely used in aromatherapy and *Lavandula stoechas*, known as French lavender, was widely used as an antiseptic and toiletry herb in ancient times by the Greeks, Romans and Arabs. To identify a plant correctly, it is necessary to at least give the generic and specific names.

There may be further divisions below this level:

- the term 'subspecies' (subsp. or ssp.) often denotes a geographical variation, for example *Lavandula stoechas* subsp. *atlantica*
- the term 'variety' (var.) indicates a rank between a botanical subspecies and forma, for example *Citrus aurantium* var. *amara*.
- the term 'forma' (f.) denotes trivial botanical differences, for example *Lavandula stoechas* f. *leucantha*
- a cultivar (given a name which is not italicised and appears in quotation marks) is a cultivated variety produced from a natural species and maintained by horticultural cultivation, for example *Lavandula angustifolia* 'Hidcote'.
- a hybrid (represented by x) is a natural or man-made cross between species, for example *Mentha* x *piperata* is a cross between *Mentha aquatica* and *Mentha spicata*.
- chemotypes (named by placing ct. followed by the chemical constituent after the name) are visually identical plants with significantly different chemical constituents and so have different therapeutic qualities.

Essential oils for therapeutic use should be labelled to indicate the above information. When buying oils, good labelling is one thing that may denote a good supplier.

ACTIVITY

Look at the labelling of oils from a selection of suppliers. Check that they use the full botanical name and give an expiry date. What other information is supplied?

Categories of oils
There are a number of ways of classifying essential oils.

By their volatility rate
Essential oils can be classified by their volatility rate – that is how quickly they evaporate into the air.

Top notes evaporate the fastest, act quickly and tend to be stimulating, for example: lemon and other citrus oils.
Middle notes evaporate more slowly and are most often used to help the general metabolism, for example: geranium and other floral and fruity oils.
Base notes evaporate slowly and are relaxing and sedating, for example: sandalwood.

Some therapists will take this into account when mixing a blend of oils, using a base note oil to hold and 'fix' a top note oil. If you smell a mixture of oils containing different 'notes', you will smell the top notes first followed by the middle and base notes.

By the Eastern Yin and Yang philosophy
The terms 'Yin' and 'Yang' are descriptions of opposite 'energies' or qualities. Yin describes cool, moist, calming, feminine qualities (e.g. rose and geranium) whereas Yang describes hot, dry, stimulating, masculine

qualities (e.g. juniper). Many oils fall between these extremes and the nearer they are to the middle the more 'balancing' they will be (e.g. sandalwood). Some therapists take this into account when selecting oils for a particular client and when deciding what effects they need to produce, whether calming, balancing or stimulating.

By the chemical constituents of the oils

An understanding of the chemistry of essential oils is important because it helps the therapist to understand their behaviour and uses. The chemistry of essential oils is complex. Some of the components are present in only minute quantities and so are hard to detect and measure. Essential oils are largely composed of volatile chemicals which are sensitive to the effects of air, light and moisture. Most contain many components with one or two major ones (e.g. peppermint is 40% menthol).

The constituents of the oils can be divided into two categories, the hydrocarbons and the oxygenated compounds.

1   Hydrocarbons consist of only hydrogen and carbon atoms arranged in a chain. The hydrocarbons found in essential oils are known as terpenes and there are two classes:
    ◆ monoterpenes ('mono' means 1) with 10 carbon atoms (e.g. camphene, pinene, limonene and carene) which occur widely in essential oils and are very prone to deteriorate if exposed to the air
    ◆ sesquiterpenes ('sesqui' means 1½) with 15 carbon atoms (e.g. chamazulene and caryophyllene) which have stronger odours and are less likely to oxidate when exposed to the air.
2   Oxygenated compounds are very diverse in chemical character and the family of oxygenated constituents includes members of many different types including those shown in Table 10.4.

Essential oils	Oygenated compound	Chemical type
Geranium, rose, palmarosa	Geraniol	Alcohols (monoterpenic)
Sandalwood	Santalolol	Alcohols (sesquiterpenic)
Black pepper, nutmeg	Eugenol	Phenols
Lemon grass, petitgrain, citronella oils	Citral	Aldehydes
Jasmine, benzoin	Benzyl acetate	Esters
Bergamot	Beragptene	Lactones (includes furocoumarins)
Jasmine, neroli	Jasmone	Ketones
Eucalyptus, rosemary, tea tree oils	Cineole	Oxides

Table 10.4 *Some of the types of oxygenated compounds found in essential oils*

Oils contain chemicals in varying proportions and tend to be classified according to which of the chemicals is predominant Table 10.5 (page 184) places these chemicals according to their general Yin or Yang qualities and describes their general effects.

YIN (calming)

Aldehydes – anti-inflammatory, antiseptic, anti-rheumatic, very calming and soothing.

Esters – the most widespread group of chemicals found in essential oils; anti-spasmodic, anti-inflammatory, anti-parasitic, cooling and soothing.

Ketones – healing, good for skin and scars, sedative, loosen mucous and soften fat so often used for people with bronchitis and cellulite. *(Ketones should not be used for too long or in high concentrations when they may be toxic).*

Sesquiterpenes – anti-inflammatory, anti-allergic, anti-parasitic; good for people with heart conditions and asthma.

—————————— Balancing line ——————————

Sesquialcohols – act as a general tonic.

Terpenes – antiseptic and anti-inflammatory; they can help to improve the blood and lymphatic circulation.

Alcohols – germicidal; some are very stimulating, but others are much less so.

Oxides – expectorant and decongestant, helping people to cough. Some are anti-parasitic, anti-viral and antiseptic.

Phenols – anti-bacterial, anti-viral, anti-fungal and anti-parasitic. *(Oils in the phenol category are very stimulating and are never used in aromatherapy massage.)*

YANG (stimulating)

Table 10.5 *The properties of essential oils*

Selecting oils for use

The selection of oils for use with a particular client is the most important part of aromatherapy and can be very daunting for the beginner.

When starting, select from a limited list – 8 to10 oils should be enough, growing to 15, to 20 and to 30 as experience increases. In the selection you choose, include more calming and balancing oils than stimulating oils. Select the more commonly used oils and be guided by a good supplier. Make sure that you know whether any of the oils have any contraindications or can have harmful effects.

ACTIVITY

Look through some lists of oils from a variety of suppliers and try to select 10 to 20 of the most useful oils to begin to use.

The following oils are those recommended by the AOC as the minimum to be studied. They are arranged alphabetically by their common names.

Basil (Ocimum basilicum)

Source	Europe, Egypt, Hungary, USA
Method of production	Steam distillation from leaves and flowers of plant
Note	Top
Aroma	Sweet, light, herbal
Key words	Steadying, clearing
Blends well with	Bergamot, geranium
Main chemical constituents	Alcohols 50–70%, ethers 5–30%, some oxides and terpenes
Uses	Steadying, good for nervous clients, good for muscle aches and pains and for coughs and colds
Precautions	Not to be used during pregnancy

Table 10.6

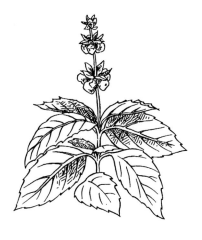

Figure 10.3 *Basil*

Benzoin (Styrax benzoin)

Source	South-east Asia, China
Method of production	The resin is gathered by tapping the tree trunk. This is then treated with an alcohol solvent to produce a resinoid which may be used like an essential oil
Note	Base to middle
Aroma	Sweet, balsamic
Key words	Soothing, clearing
Blends well with	Cypress, juniper, lemon, rose, sandalwood, other spicy oils
Main chemical constituents	Esters 70%, acids, aldehydes
Uses	Good for colds and catarrh, helps to clear phlegm from chest, also rheumatic pain and chapped skin, very calming
Precautions	None known

Table 10.7

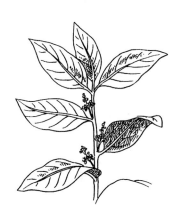

Figure 10.4 *Benzoin*

Bergamot (*Citrus aurantium bergamia*)

Source	Italy, Sicily, tropical Africa, Asia
Method of production	Cold expression from the rind of the fruit of the bitter orange while it is still green and unripe
Note	Top
Aroma	Fruity, sweet
Key words	Uplifting
Blends well with	Basil, frankincense, geranium, lavender, neroli, sandalwood, ylang ylang, other citrus oils
Main chemical constituents	Esters 30–65%, terpenes, alcohols. Substances known as furocumarins are also present and are resposible for the oil being photosensitising. Bergamot oil can be purchased which has had the furocumarins removed
Uses	Uplifting, good for people who are anxious or depressed and having difficulty sleeping. Calming and good for the digestion
Precautions	Bergomot has been shown to sensitise skin to ultraviolet light so do not use within 3 hours of going out into the sun or using a sunbed. Should not be used on children.

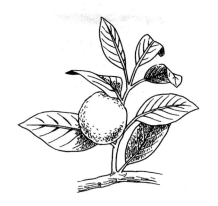

Figure 10.5 *Bergamot*   **Table 10.8**

Black pepper (*Piper nigrum*)

Source	Southern India, Malaysia, China, Madagascar
Method of production	Steam distillation of the dried unripe fruit
Note	Middle
Aroma	Spicy, fresh, peppery
Key words	Stimulating, digestive
Blends well with	Frankincense, lavender, rosemary, sandalwood, other spicy oils
Main chemical constituents	Monoterpenes 70–90%, sesquiterpenes 10–30%, traces of alcohols, ketones
Uses	Stimulating, good for the circulation and conditions related to poor circulation, can stimulate the appetite. Warming and good for chesty colds, expectorant
Precautions	None known

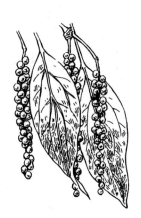

Figure 10.6 *Black pepper*   **Table 10.9**

Cedarwood (*Cedrus atlantica*)

Source	North Africa, Algeria, Morocco
Method of production	Steam distillation of the wood obtained from the Atlas cedar tree
Note	Middle
Aroma	Camphorous, sweet, balsamic
Key words	Toning, respiration
Blends well with	Bergamot, clary sage, frankincense, ylang ylang
Main chemical constituents	Sesquiterpenes 50%, sesquialcohols 20–30%, ketones
Uses	Good for water retention, cellulite, has a general tonic effect and is good for oily skin. Repels insects
Precautions	None known

Table 10.10

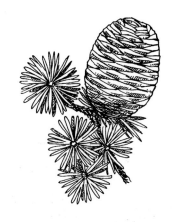

Figure 10.7 *Cedar*

There are a number of oils known as chamomile, including German chamomile, Roman chamomile and Moroccan chamomile which are considered here.

German chamomile (*Matricaria recutita*, also known as *Chamomilla recutita*)

Source	Europe, Asia
Method of production	Steam distillation of the flower
Note	Middle to base
Aroma	Fruity, sharp
Key words	Allergies, skin
Blends well with	Benzoin, clary sage, geranium, lavender, citrus oils
Main chemical constituents	Oxides 30–50%, terpenes 30%, alcohols up to 60%
Uses	Very useful for spasmodic or inflammatory conditions. It is also good for allergies, relieves pain and is good for the skin
Precautions	Use in low concentration, has been known to cause sensitisation

Table 10.11

Figure 10.8 *German chamomile*

Roman chamomile (*Chamaemelum nobile* also known as *Anthemis nobilis*)

Source	Europe, North America
Method of production	Steam distillation from the flowers
Note	Middle to top
Aroma	Warm, fruity like hay
Key words	Soothing
Blends well with	Benzoin, clary sage, geranium, lavender, patchouli, vetiver, citrus oils
Main chemical constituents	Esters 70–80%, ketones, alcohols. Azulene is responsible for the bluish colour of the oil
Uses	Anti-spasmodic and anti-inflammatory. Good for skin irritations, muscular pain and is excellent for treating stressed clients
Precautions	None known

Table 10.12

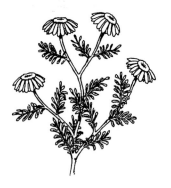

Figure 10.9 *Roman chamomile*

Moroccan chamomile (*Ormenis mixta* also *Ormenis multicaulis*)

Source	Northern Africa, southern Spain
Method of production	Steam distillation from the flowers
Note	Top
Aroma	Fresh, flowery, balsamic
Key words	Uplifting
Blends well with	Cedarwood, cypress, lavender, vetiver
Main chemical constituents	Monoterpenes 50–60%, alcohols 30%, oxides, esters
Uses	Antibacterial and anti-inflammatory, it is good for skin conditions especially acne. It is also uplifting and good for headaches
Precautions	Avoid during pregnancy

Table 10.13

Clary sage (*Salvia sclarea*)

Source	Europe, Middle East, USA
Method of production	Steam distillation of the flowers
Note	Middle to top
Aroma	Slightly spicy, warm, a little camphorous
Key words	Relaxing
Blends well with	Blends well with citrus oils, chamomile, geranium, juniper, lavender, ylang ylang
Main chemical constituents	Esters 75%, alcohols 20%, terpenes, oxides, ketones
Uses	Good for exhaustion and overwork, a good muscle relaxant, anti-depressant. Known as a uterine tonic
Precautions	Not to be used during pregnancy or the menopause

Table 10.14

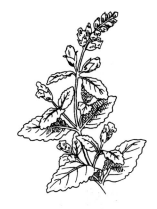

Figure 10.10 *Clary sage*

Cypress (*Cupressus sempervirens*)

Source	Mediterranean region, France, Spain, Morocco
Method of production	Steam distillation of the leaves, twigs and cones
Note	Top, middle and base
Aroma	Fresh and piney
Key words	Diuretic
Blends well with	Benzoin, bergamot, chamomile, frankincense, juniper, lavender, lemon, tea tree, other woody oils
Main chemical constituents	Terpenes 70%, alcohols 10–15%, aldehydes
Uses	Stimulates the circulation, good for rheumatic pain, menopausal problems, cellulite, coughs and colds
Precautions	None known

Table 10.15

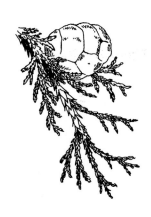

Figure 10.11 *Cypress*

There are a number of eucalyptus oils used in aromatherapy. Common eucalyptus (*Eucalyptus globulus*), and lemon-scented eucalyptus also known as lemon gum (*Eucalyptus citriodora*) are considered here. *Eucalyptus radiata* ct. cineole is similar in most respects to *Eucalyptus globulus* but is more gentle in its aroma and effects.

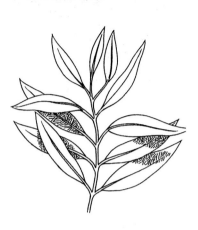

Figure 10.12 *Eucalyptus*

Common eucalyptus (*Eucalyptus globulus*)

Source	Originally Australia, now also Spain, Portugal, USA, Brazil, China
Method of production	Steam distillation of the leaf
Note	Top
Aroma	Strong, balsamic, camphorous
Key words	Respiratory
Blends well with	Renzoin, frankincense, lavender, peppermint, tea tree, thyme
Main chemical constituents	Oxides 70–90%, terpenes 10–20%, alcohols
Uses	Decongestant in helping people with colds or bronchitis to cough, also relieves muscular or rheumatic pain. Very useful as an inhalant
Precautions	None known

Table 10.16

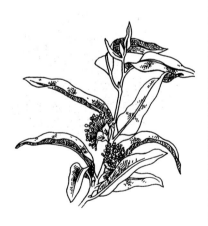

Figure 10.13 *Lemon-scented eucalyptus, lemon gum*

Lemon-scented eucalyptus or lemon gum (*Eucalyptus citriadora*)

Source	Australia, Brazil, China, Southern Africa
Method of production	Method of production steam distillation of the leaf
Note	Top
Aroma	Lemon-like, camphorous
Key words	Cooling
Blends well with	Benzoin, frankincense, lavender, tea tree, thyme
Main chemical constituents	Aldehydes 60–70%, alcohols 20%, esters
Uses	Cooling, anti-infectious, good for rheumatic conditions. Used as an insect repellent
Precautions	None known

Table 10.17

Fennel (*Foeniculum vulgare*)

Source	Europe, India, Japan, USA
Method of production	Steam distillation of the crushed seeds
Note	Middle
Aroma	Aniseed-like, pungent
Key words	Digestive
Blends well with	Geranium, lavender, sandalwood, other oils from seeds
Main chemical constituents	Phenols 50–70%, terpenes, alcohols, oxides
Uses	Mainly used for digestive problems, it is also a diuretic
Precautions	Not to be used on pregnant or breast-feeding mothers, on young children or anyone suffering from disease of the uterus. Do not use on damaged skin and only use a 1% solution

Table 10.18

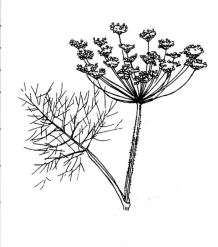

Figure 10.14 *Fennel*

Frankincense (*Boswellia carteri*)

Source	Middle East, North Africa, Arabia, China
Method of production	Steam distillation of the gum which is obtained by making incisions in the surface of the tree trunk to allow a milky resin to collect. This resin hardens to form the gum on exposure to air.
Note	Base
Aroma	Balsamic, camphorous
Key words	Stress-relieving
Blends well with	Basil, bergamot, black pepper, citrus oils, lavender, sandalwood, vetiver
Main chemical constituents	Terpenes 50%, alcohols, ketones, oxides
Uses	Rejuvenating, very good on older skins, good for chest conditions especially stress-related ones, calming and anti-inflammatory
Precautions	None known

Table 10.19

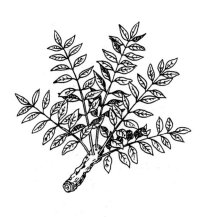

Figure 10.15 *Frankincense*

Geranium (*Pelargonium graveolens*)

Source	France, Italy, South Africa, Réunion Island, Spain
Method of production	Steam distillation of the leaves
Note	Middle
Aroma	Floral, spicy
Key words	Balancing
Blends well with	Alcohols 75%, Esters 10–15%, ketones, aldehydes
Main chemical constituents	Most oils especially basil, bergamot, chamomile, lavender, patchouli, citrus
Uses	Healing oil for skin disorders, bruises and burns. Anti-inflammatory and good for respiratory and digestive conditions, balancing. Good for dry and red skins, it stimulates the lymphatic system and can be useful for cellulite.
Precautions	None known

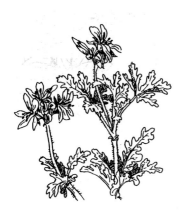

Figure 10.16 *Geranium*   **Table 10.20**

Ginger (*Zingiber officinalis*)

Source	West Indies, West Africa, India, Malaysia, Australia
Method of production	Steam distillation of the ginger 'root' which is in fact an underground stem or rhizome
Note	Top, middle and base all present
Aroma	Very spicy and pungent
Key words	Warming
Blends well with	Benzoin, cedar, frankincense, sandalwood, citrus oils
Main chemical constituents	Terpenes 55%, alcohols, aldehydes, ketones
Uses	Very warming and decongesting, used for nausea and aching muscles
Precautions	None known

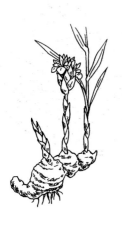

Figure 10.17 *Ginger*   **Table 10.21**

Grapefruit (*Citrus paradisi*)

Source	Brazil, California, Florida, Mediterranean countries, Israel
Method of production	Cold expression from the rind of the fruit
Note	Top
Aroma	Light, citrus
Key words	Uplifting
Blends well with	Clary sage, eucalyptus, geranium, juniper, lavender, rosemary, tea tree, other citrus oils
Main chemical constituents	Terpenes 95%, aldehydes
Uses	Stimulates the lymphatic and digestive systems, calming and uplifting
Precautions	Phototoxic, exposure to sunlight or sunbeds within 12 hours may lead to patchy discoloration of the skin

Table 10.22

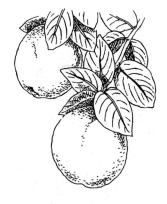

Figure 10.18 *Grapefruit*

Jasmine (*Jasminum officinale*)

Source	India, Egypt, North Africa, Turkey, Japan, China
Method of production	An absolute is obtained by solvent extraction from the flowers, or pure essential oil may be obtained by traditional enfleurage. This makes it a very expensive oil
Note	Top to middle
Aroma	Very sweet, floral
Key words	Emotional
Blends well with	Bergamot, cypress, lavender, sandalwood, ylang ylang
Main chemical constituents	Aldehydes 45%, alcohols
Uses	Calming and anti-depressive, useful for insomnia and nervous tension
Precautions	Not to be used in pregnancy although jasmine is sometimes used to help during labour

Table 10.23

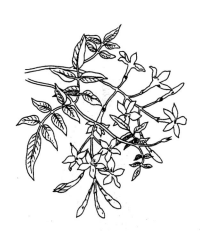

Figure 10.19 *Jasmine*

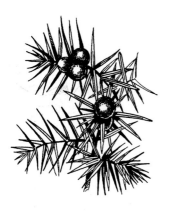

Figure 10.20 *Juniper*

Juniper (*Juniperus communis*)

Source	Northern Europe, Asia, USA, Siberia
Method of production	Steam distillation of the ripe berries
Note	Top to middle
Aroma	Woody, fresh, piney
Key words	Cleansing
Blends well with	Cypress, lavender, rosemary, citrus oils
Main chemical constituents	Terpenes 90–95%, alcohols
Uses	Diuretic, good for people with fluid retention or cellulite and can be helpful in cases of cystitis. Good on some problem skins for such as acne, can be used as a disinfectant
Precautions	Not to be used in cases of kidney disorders

Table 10.24

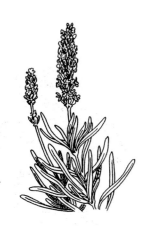

Figure 10.21 *Lavender*

Lavender (*Lavandula angustifolia* or *Lavandula officinalis*)

Source	Mediterranean countries, Bulgaria, Russia, Croatia, England
Method of production	Steam distillation of the flowers
Note	Middle
Aroma	Floral, sweet
Key words	Immune system
Blends well with	Floral and citrus oils, bergamot, chamomile, clary sage, geranium, lemon, peppermint, pine, tea tree
Main chemical constituents	Esters 35–55%, alcohols 30–50%, terpenes, oxides
Uses	Boosts the immune system, calming, balancing, healing especially burns, muscular pain, problem skins. The most versatile, useful oil
Precautions	None known. Take care to select the correct oil, there are many different oils sold under the name 'Lavender'

Table 10.25

Lemon (*Citrus limon*)

Source	Mediterranean countries, Florida, California, Australia, Brazil
Method of production	Cold expression of the rind of the ripe fruit
Note	Top
Aroma	Light, citrus, slightly sour
Key words	Stimulating, refreshing
Blends well with	Benzoin, cedar, eucalyptus, fennel, juniper, lavender, ylang ylang
Main chemical constituents	Terpenes 50–90%, aldehydes
Uses	Useful for clients recovering from viral-type illnesses, also to stimulate the circulation so useful over areas of fat and cellulite and in rheumatic conditions, refreshing
Precautions	Phototoxic so avoid exposure to sunlight or sunbeds for 12 hours, can cause skin irritation so needs to be used in very low dosage. Do not use during pregnancy

Table 10.26

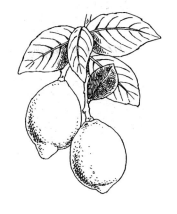

Figure 10.22 *Lemon*

Lemongrass (*Cymbopogon citratus*)

Source	India, the Far East, West Indies, Sri Lanka
Method of production	Steam distillation of the grass after it has been finely chopped
Note	Top
Aroma	Strong, lemon-like, sweet
Key words	Strengthening
Blends well with	Bergamot, cypress, lavender, lemon
Main chemical constituents	Aldehydes 75%–90%, terpenes
Uses	Strengthening, good for muscle aches and pains, stomach upsets fungal skin infections such as athlete's foot
Precautions	Not to be used on children or on people with broken or hypersensitive skin. Only use in 1% solution or less

Table 10.27

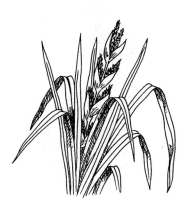

Figure 10.23 *Lemongrass*

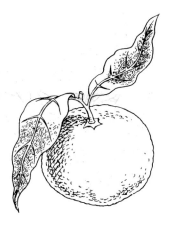

Figure 10.24 *Mandarin orange*

Table 10.28

Mandarin orange (*Citrus reticulata*)

Source	Greece, Spain, North Africa, Italy, Florida, California
Method of production	Cold expression of the rind of the fruit
Note	Middle
Aroma	Sweet, light citrus
Key words	Calming, insomnia
Blends well with	Bergamot, clary sage, geranium, lavender, lemon, marjoram, sandalwood, ylang ylang, all the spicy oils
Main chemical constituents	Terpenes 95%, alcohols
Uses	Calming, good for insomnia and nervous tension, soothing for stomach cramps and indigestion
Precautions	May be phototoxic; avoid exposure to sunlight after application

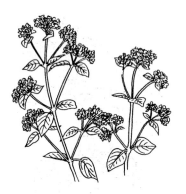

Figure 10.25 *Marjoram (sweet)*

Table 10.29

Marjoram (sweet) (*Origanum marjorana*)

Source	Bulgaria, Hungary, North Africa, France, Egypt
Method of production	Steam distillation of the whole flowering herb
Note	Middle to base
Aroma	Sweet, woody, herbaceous
Key words	Analgesic
Blends well with	Bergamot, cedar, chamomile, eucalyptus, lavender, neroli, tea tree
Main chemical constituents	Alcohols 50%, terpenes 30%, esters
Uses	Warming and ant-spasmodic, it is very useful for the digestive and respiratory systems and also as an analgesic in arthritic conditions and muscular pains
Precautions	None known

Neroli (orange blossom) (*Citrus aurantium* var. *amara*)

Source	Mediterranean countries, West Indies, California, Haiti
Method of production	Steam distillation of the flowers of the bitter orange. Yield is low and this is an expensive oil
Note	Middle
Aroma	Floral, rich, orange-like
Key words	Stress
Blends well with	Other citrus oils, chamomile, clary sage, geranium, lavender, lemon grass, marjoram, sandalwood
Main chemical constituents	Alcohols 40%, terpenes 35%, esters, aldehydes
Uses	Good for fatigue, aids sleep, anti-depressive, antibacterial, good for the digestive system
Precautions	None known

Table 10.30

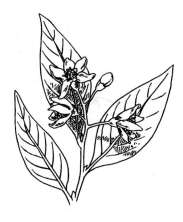

Figure 10.26 *Neroli (orange blossom)*

Patchouli (*Pogostemon cablin*)

Source	Malaysia, Philippines, China, India
Method of production	Steam distillation of the dried leaves
Note	Base
Aroma	Oriental, spicy, musky
Key words	Infection, skin
Blends well with	Bergamot, cedar, lavender, sandalwood, ylang ylang
Main chemical constituents	Sesquiterpenes 50%, alcohols 45%, ketones, oxides
Uses	Anti-inflammatory, good for skin infections, acne, digestive system, nausea, also acts as an insect repellent
Precautions	None known

Table 10.31

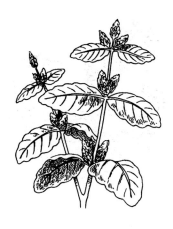

Figure 10.27 *Patchouli*

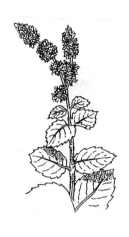

Figure 10.28 *Peppermint*

Peppermint (*Mentha piperita*)

Source	All temperate zones
Method of production	Steam distillation of the leaves
Note	Top to middle
Aroma	Fresh, cool, minty
Key words	Cooling
Blends well with	Benzoin, eucalyptus, geranium, lavender, lemon, rosemary
Main chemical constituents	Alcohols 50%, ketones 40%, oxides, terpenes
Uses	Cooling, traditionally used for stomach upsets, also for clearing the head and for coughs and colds. Very good for tired feet.
Precautions	Avoid during pregnancy and breast-feeding and on children under the age of 5. Avoid using on people with heart disease or epilepsy. Can irritate sensitive skins.

Table 10.32

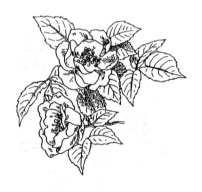

Figure 10.29 *Rose otto*

Rose otto (*Rosa damascena*)

Source	Bulgaria, Turkey, Morocco, India
Method of production	Steam distillation of the flower petals. This gives a low yield and the oil is very expensive
Note	Middle
Aroma	Floral, sweet, rich
Key words	Antidepressant
Blends well with	Bergamot, chamomile, clary sage, geranium, jasmine, lavender, patchouli sandalwood, ylang ylang
Main chemical constituents	Alcohols 60–80%, terpenes 20–25%, esters
Uses	Good for anxiety and depression, insomnia, menstrual problems and pain
Precautions	Oils sold as 'Rose' are often adulterated

Table 10.33

Rosemary (*Rosemarinus officinalis* ct. cineole)

Source	Mediterranean countries, Middle East, California
Method of production	Steam distillation of the flowering twigs
Note	Top to middle
Aroma	Camphorous, woody
Key words	Stimulating
Blends well with	Basil, citrus oils, frankincense, lemon grass, peppermint, tea tree, thyme
Main chemical constituents	Oxides 20–55% terpenes 10–35%, ketones 5-30%
Uses	Uplifting, useful for people with colds or other respiratory problems. Good for stiffness and discomfort in the muscles. After lavender, this is the most commonly used oil.
Precautions	Rosemary is contraindicated in pregnant, breast-feeding or epileptic clients and in those with high blood pressure. It should not be used for too long a period as it can be stimulating.

Table 10.34

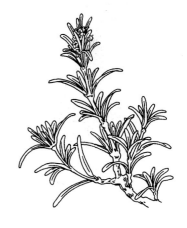

Figure 10.30 *Rosemary*

Sandalwood (*Santalum album*)

Source	India
Method of production	Steam distillation of the heartwood of the tree
Note	Base
Aroma	Woody, balsamic, musky
Key words	Balancing
Blends well with	Benzoin, black pepper, bergamot, geranium, lavender, lemon, patchouli
Main chemical constituents	Sesquialcohols 70%, terpenes 20%
Uses	Balancing, good on the skin, for stress-related conditions, nervous tension and chest conditions
Precautions	None known

Table 10.35

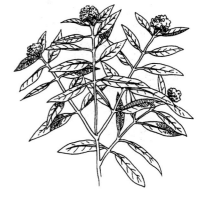

Figure 10.31 *Sandalwood*

Tea tree (*Melaleuca alternifolia*)

Source	New South Wales, Australia
Method of production	Steam distillation of the leaf and twigs
Note	Top
Aroma	Strongly medicinal, spicy
Key words	Antiseptic
Blends well with	Bergamot, cypress, frankincense, lavender, rosemary
Main chemical constituents	Alcohols and sesquialcohols 70–80%, terpenes and sesquiterpenes 20%, oxides
Uses	One of the best known of the essential oils and now being incorporated into creams and soaps for its anti-fungal, anti-bacterial and anti-viral qualities, particularly in helping fungal conditions such as thrush and athlete's foot. It seems to stimulate the immune system and is particularly valuable if a cold or flu might be developing
Precautions	May cause irritation on sensitive skins

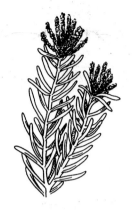

Figure 10.32 *Tea tree*

Table 10.36

Thyme (sweet) (*Thymus vulgaris* ct. thymol)

Source	All temperate zones especially France and Spain
Method of production	Steam distillation of the leaves and flowers
Note	Top and middle, some base
Aroma	Herbaceous, pungent, medicinal
Key words	Antiseptic
Blends well with	Bergamot, lavender, lemon, pine, rosemary
Main chemical constituents	Phenols 30–40%, alcohols 15–20%, terpenes
Uses	Anti-bacterial and antiseptic for acne and skin infections, warming for stiff joints, general tonic
Precautions	Avoid in pregnancy, breast-feeding, and children under 5. Use in dilution of no more than 1% and do not use on sensitive skin

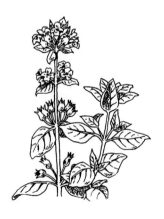

Figure 10.33 *Thyme*

Table 10.37

Ylang ylang (*Cananga odorata*)

Source	Madagascar, Philippines, Indonesia
Method of production	Steam distillation of freshly picked flowers
Note	Middle to base
Aroma	Very sweet, floral, spicy
Key words	Warming, aphrodisiac
Blends well with	Bergamot, clary sage, jasmine, neroli, rose, sandalwood
Main chemical constituents	Alcohols and sesquialcohols 30%, terpenes up to 50%, esters
Uses	Anti-depressive, warming, soothes and boosts confidence, traditionally known as an aphrodisiac
Precautions	None known

Table 10.38

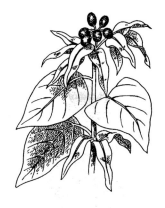

Figure 10.34 *Ylang ylang*

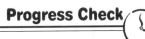

Progress Check

Check that you remember the main effects of each of the chemical categories.

- Aldehydes
- Esters
- Ketones
- Monoterpenic alcohols
- Oxides
- Phenols
- Sesquiterpenes
- Sesquiterpenic alcohols
- Terpenes

There are some other useful essential oils. The effects for which they are best known are listed here.

Aniseed (**Pimpinella anisum**)

- Note: middle
- Main chemical constituent: ester
- Uses: warming, antiseptic, expectorant
- Precautions: Avoid using on sensitive skin especially allergic or inflamed skin

Immortelle (**Helichrysum angustifolium**)

- Note: middle
- Main chemical constituent: ketone
- Uses: expectorant, good for aches and pains, skin conditions, breaks in the skin
- Blends well with: chamomile, clary sage, geranium, lavender

Myrrh (**Commiphora myrrha**)

- Note: base
- Main chemical constituent: sesquiterpene
- Uses: healing, good for the chest, sedative
- Blends well with: frankincense, sandalwood, benzoin, juniper
- Precautions: not to be used during pregnancy

Myrtle (**Myrtis communis**)

- Note: middle
- Main chemical constituent: oxide
- Uses: good for catarrh, slightly sedative, soothing
- Blends well with: bergamot, lavender, rosemary, clary sage

Petitgrain (**Citrus aurantium** *subsp.* **amara**)

- Note: top and middle
- Main chemical constituent: ester
- Uses: calming, good for digestive and nervous disorders
- Blends well with: other citrus oils, sandalwood, chamomile, rosemary

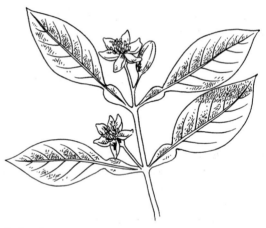

Figure 10.35 *Petitgrain*

Pine (**Pinus sylvestris**)

- Note: middle
- Main chemical constituent: terpene
- Uses: good for colds and chest infections, stimulating
- Blends well with: tea tree, rosemary, lavender, juniper
- Precautions: avoid in allergic skin conditions

Vetiver (**Vetiveria zizanoides**)

- Note: middle
- Main chemical constituent: sesquialcohol
- Uses: calming, stimulates the circulatory system
- Blends well with: sandalwood, patchouli, lavender, clary sage

Chemical variations within species

Some of these oils may have 'ct.' after the full name on the label which stands for 'chemotype'. This is a term applied to plants of the same genus and species but which differ in their chemical composition, this

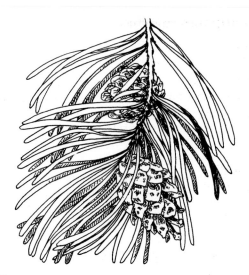

Figure 10.36 *Pine*

in turn affects their therapeutic use. These differences may occur as a result of:

- cross pollination and can occur in the wild
- the place and manner of growing
- genetic and environmental factors.

The following are some examples of different chemotypes within a species.

Thyme

- *Thymus vulgaris* ct. thymol: this thyme is strongly antiseptic and aggressive to the skin as thymol is a phenol. Harvested in the spring the oil will contain 30% thymol and in the autumn 60–70% thymol.
- *Thymus vulgaris* ct. carvacrol: this thyme behaves the same way as ct. thymol but the phenol is carvacol. This also is 30% in spring and 60–80% in autumn.

These two thymes are sometimes called 'red thyme' and are major anti-infective agents.

The rest of the thymes are alcohol-containing types, sometimes called yellow or sweet thymes.

- *Thymus vulgaris* ct. linalol: much gentler but also anti-bacterial and anti-fungal.
- *Thymus vulgaris* ct. thujanol 4: does not show seasonal variation, contains 50% alcohol, cannot be cultivated, is said to stimulate the immune system, is neurotonic, and hormone-like.
- *Thymus vulgaris* ct. terpineol: contains the ester, terpenyl acetate (more in the spring) and the alcohol terpineol. This type of thyme is much safer on the skin than the red thymes.
- *Thymus vulgaris* ct. geraniol: contains the ester geranyl acetate and 80–90% of the alcohol geraniol. There is a seasonal variation. The geraniol gives it a lemony smell. It is anti-viral, anti-fungal, neurotonic and cardiotonic.

[Source: *Aromatherapy for Health Professionals*, S. Price and L. Price, published by Churchill Livingstone, 1995)

Rosemary

💧 *Rosmarinus officinalis* ct. camphor: contains 30% camphor, stimulates the circulatory system, is mucolytic (it loosens mucus), a decongestant and a muscle relaxant.

💧 *Rosmarinus officinalis* ct. cineole: contains 40–50% cineole, is anti-fungal, anti-bacterial and mucolytic.

💧 *Rosmarinus officinalis* ct. verbenone: contains 15-40% verbenone, is mucolytic, an expectorant, an anti-spasmodic and it also may help to regulate the endocrine system.

Some other oils with different chemotypes are tarragon, basil, sage and melissa.

ACTIVITY

Look through the uses of the above oils and select those oils which may be considered Yin oils and those which might be Yang.

Progress Check

1 What is an essential oil?
2 Give five factors governing the quality of essential oils.

Key Terms

You need to know what these words mean. Go back through the chapter or check in the glossary to find out.

💧 absolute
💧 anti-inflammatory
💧 antiseptic
💧 base note
💧 chemotype
💧 concrete
💧 distillation
💧 diuretic
💧 expectorant
💧 expression
💧 middle note
💧 solvent
💧 subspecies
💧 top note
💧 volatile

USING THE OILS

After working through this chapter you will be able to:
- describe the qualities of a number of carrier oils
- select the amounts of carrier and essential oils for massage
- explain the principles of blending and synergy
- relate the consultation process to treatment planning
- prepare a plan for an aromatherapy treatment
- select oils which blend together well for aromatherapy massage
- consider further ways of using essential oils other than for massage.

Essential oils are very concentrated and should never be used undiluted on the skin. For an aromatherapy massage they must be mixed with a carrier oil which will provide lubrication for the massage as well as carrying the therapeutic essential oils being used.

Carrier oils

Although mineral oils such as baby oil are sometimes used for massage, they are not suitable as carrier oils as they are not easily absorbed by the skin. You can use any vegetable oil so long as it is fairly light and does not have a strong smell which would overpower the essential oils. Just as a good cook will insist that the olive oil they use should be of the finest quality, so an aromatherapist will use only carrier oils that are organically grown, unrefined and cold-pressed. This will preserve any beneficial vitamins or minerals. Again, the advice of a reputable supplier is invaluable.

The carrier oil chosen can be used on its own with the essential oils or can have small amounts of other carrier oils mixed with them. When beginning to mix oils, grapeseed oil is probably best used as a carrier oil as it is easily available and not expensive. Sweet almond oil is also an excellent choice. Other oils may be mixed with the carrier oils in small amounts before blending in the essential oils. Those containing gamma-linolenic acid (GLA) are particularly good for the skin.

All vegetable carrier oils will become rancid (oxidise) after being exposed to the air for some time, so relatively small amounts should be bought at one time and only small quantities should be mixed at a time to avoid wasting essential oils.

There are other oils used such as hazelnut, camellia, macademia nut, cashew nut, olive oil and safflower oil. Personal preference influences the choice of carrier oils but the most commonly used in the UK is probably sweet almond oil.

Oil	Properties	Cost	Uses
Almond (sweet)	Clear pale yellow, nearly odourless, good lubricant, nourishing to the skin, fairly stable	Average	Commonly used on the body and face, good for dry skin and eczema
Apricot kernel	Pale orange, slightly sticky, stable, vitamin A, nourishing	Average	Good for dry and ageing skin, especially the face
Avocado	Dark green, rich and heavy, fair stability with slightly pungent smell. Contains essential fatty acids and vitamins A and D, very nourishing, easily absorbed	Above average	Used only as a supplement to other carrier oils e.g. 5–10 % of a carrier oil for use on a very dry or ageing skin
Borage	Golden colour, strong smell unless deodorised. Poor stability. Rich in vitamins, minerals and GLA (23 %)	Expensive	5–10 % additive to other carrier oils. Improves elasticity and hydration of the skin. Good for psoriasis, eczema and prematurely aged skin
Coconut	Colourless, sweet, permeates well	Above average	Must be used 50:50 with another oil to prevent it solidifying
Evening primrose	Golden, poor stability, 7–9 % GLA, vitamin E. Regenerative and anti-inflammatory	Expensive	5–10 % additive particularly good for prematurely aged skins, eczema, psoriasis and allergies
Grapeseed	Pale green, light and thin, high in polyunsaturates, penetrates well, very stable	Inexpensive	Good for body massage, slightly astringent so good for oily skin or acne
Jojoba	Fine, golden, penetrates well, anti-inflammatory	Expensive	Good for dry, sensitive skin, eczema, psoriasis and allergies
Peach kernel	Rich, light stable, has vitamins A and E and essential fatty acids. Nourishes and penetrates well	Average	Good for itching, dry skin, excellent for facial massage
Rosa rubiginosa	High in GLA and essential fatty acids. Is a cell regenerator	Expensive	5–10 % additive for dry, peeling, cracked or devitalised skin, also infected, blotchy or hyper pigmented skin, scars
Soya bean	Pale, light, stable, penetrates well, high in polyunsaturates and vitamin E	Inexpensive	Easy to use in body and face massage
Sunflower	Golden, fairly rich, poor stability, fair penetration	Average	Body and face massage
Wheatgerm	Deep amber, rich, fairly thick, stable, pungent smell. Has vitamins A and E and 80 % unsaturated fatty acids	Above average	10–20 % addition to body and face especially for dry, mature skin, stretch marks or scar tissue. Works as an anti-oxidant preventing other oils from going rancid

Table 11.1 *Properties and uses of some carrier oils*

Mixing the oils for aromatherapy massage

It is usual in an aromatherapy massage to use two or three essential oils in a carrier oil, blended together for use in the massage. When two or more essential oils are mixed, they blend together to produce effects which are more than the combined effects of each oil. Some oils blend together better than others and enhance each other's effects. This synergic effect allows oils to be blended for the benefit of the individual client. The synergy of the oils should be considered when selecting oils to be blended together.

To prepare a blend for massage you will need:

 ♦ a glass or clear plastic measuring bottle that is marked in millilitres
 ♦ a glass rod for stirring.

The amount of carrier oil needed for the massage is measured into the bottle and the drops of essential oils added. It is then stirred with the glass rod or shaken if there is a stopper and then it is ready for use.

Amounts of oil needed for massage will vary but a useful 'rule of thumb' for a full body massage is to allow 10 ml for a small person, 14 ml for a medium size and up to 20 ml for a large person. In women, the dress size is a good indicator.

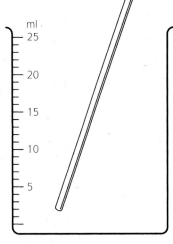

Figure 11.1 *Mixing equipment*

GOOD PRACTICE

Try not to mix too much oil as it will be wasted.

For body massage, the essential oils should form 2 % of the blend. It is not practical to measure the essential oils in millilitres as 2 % of essential oil in 10 ml of carrier oil would be 0.2 ml. The essential oils are therefore measured in drops. 1 % of essential oils in 10 ml of carrier is 2.5 drops and 2 % in 10 ml of carrier is 5 drops. So, if you divide the millilitres of carrier oil by two, the answer gives you the number of drops of essential oils to give a 2 % solution i.e. up to 5 drops of essential oils can be added to 10 ml of carrier, up to 7 drops in 14 ml and up to 10 drops in 20 ml.

For facial massage, the essential oils should form 1 % of the blend, half the strength of that used for the body.

The scalp can be treated with a 2 % or 1 %, whichever is the most convenient, and will need at least 5 ml of carrier oil as the hair tends to absorb some.

The oils selected for use are always the result of a careful consultation process which will take into account client preference and their predominant problems. One, two or three essential oils may be used to make up a blend.

Factors to be considered in making up a blend

 ♦ The choice of essential and carrier oils must be appropriate for the condition of the client.
 ♦ The fragrance of individual oils should be acceptable to the client.
 ♦ The fragrance of the mix of oils should be acceptable to the client.

- Oils with very strong fragrance (e.g. eucalyptus) should be used in small amounts so that they do not dominate.
- The oils chosen should complement each other (have synergy).

The selection and blending of oils for use with a particular client is the most important part of the aromatherapy treatment. As we have seen, some oils blend together well and are said to be acting synergistically as they seem to help each other's effects. Other oils may inhibit each others effects and do not blend so well together. If a start is made by using the oils that the client is attracted to and which fit into the category that will help the main problems the client presents, then that is an excellent start.

Examples of oils that work well together are given in the lists of essential oils (see pages 185–201, chapter 10).

SAFE PRACTICE

The same essential oil should not be used over a long period as it may become ineffective. It is wise to vary the oils from time to time.

When selecting a blend for a client, select the general categories that suit the problems, for example for a client who has worries at work and gets constant cold-like symptoms you would select:

- an ester for the cooling, soothing qualities
- an oxide to help the cold symptoms
- maybe a ketone to loosen mucus if the cold is a chesty one.

Then, from the available oils, choose the ones that the client likes and that you think will go well together, for example lavender, eucalyptus and rosemary. Experience will lead you to an instinctive blend of oils.

Consultation

Before developing a treatment plan, full consultation with the client is necessary.

ACTIVITY
Re-read chapters 3 and 10 on consultation procedures.

REMEMBER
Consultation should take into account

1 Medical background:
- contraindications
- problem areas.

2 Lifestyle

3 Personality:
- temperament
- emotional state.

The consultation process is especially important in clients attending for aromatherapy massage. This is because the effects of massage and the effects of the essential oils have to be considered.

The purpose of the consultation is to find out firstly that it is safe to treat the client and secondly how best to help the client.

The consultation procedure to establish the medical background is fully covered in chapter 3 and questions related to lifestyle and personality and to temperament and emotional state are covered in chapter 9 (page 174).

Consultation is an ongoing process which should continue throughout treatment.

With a colleague acting as a client, carry out a consultation with the aim of selecting suitable oils for the client. Ask the colleague to explain how effective the questions were in eliciting relevant information.

Treatment plan following full consultation

- Decide on the aims of treatment, focusing on the client's main and secondary problems.
- List the essential oils suitable for use with these problems.
- Select two or three compatible oils from this list.
- Ask the client to smell and approve each individual oil.
- Ask the client to smell and approve the oils together.

Decide on the treatment method:

- full body massage
- full body massage with facial massage
- part body massage.

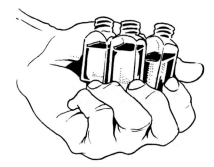

Figure 11.2 *Let the client smell the selection*

Agree time scale and charges with client

Many clients may feel uncomfortable if the therapist assumes that there will be a series of treatments. Always ask if a client wants to book a series or individual treatments.

Aromatherapy treatments will be most effective if they can be carried out quite intensively. Twice weekly is ideal to start, then reducing to once weekly. The reason for this is that the oils (with some exceptions) remain in the body for up to 72 hours so that the effects begin to wear off after 2 to 3 days. Intensive treatment will be particularly suitable for clients suffering from symptoms of stress.

> **REMEMBER**
> It is important to consider the client's availability when discussing the length and number of treatments.

Once the treatment method and time scale have been decided, the treatment plan is carried out.

Example of a treatment plan

Following full consultation with a middle-aged, female client you decide the aims of the treatment.

- To provide general relaxation (very busy, tense lifestyle).
- To improve sluggish circulation (cold hands and feet).

You advise the time scale of the treatment.

- Ideally over a period of six weeks.
- Full body aromatherapy massage every other week alternating with an aromatherapy facial or hand and foot treatment in the other weeks.

> **REMEMBER**
> Courses of treatments paid for in advance act as an incentive to the client and help the therapist.

You advise that costs are as per listed charges.

You list suitable oils to use for relaxation.

- lavender
- geranium

- Roman chamomile
- frankincense.

You list suitable oils to use to stimulate the circulation.

- rosemary
- juniper
- black pepper
- lemon.

You ask the client to smell each briefly and reject any not liked. You select two oils, one from each group, say lavender and rosemary, and let the client smell them together. If the combination is approved by the client the oils can be mixed.

- For the full body massage, in 15ml carrier mix 5 drops of lavender and 2 of rosemary.
- For the facial massage, in 6 ml of carrier oil mix 2 drops of lavender and 1 of rosemary.

More than two essential oils can be used but not more than four. If three oils are preferred for the body massage, the blend may be: 4 drops of lavender, 2 drops of rosemary and 1 drop of Roman chamomile.

Offer to mix oils or products for home use or take the opportunity to sell aromatherapy products.

REMEMBER
Check for any contraindications.

Complementary home care advice

Complementary home care advice should be given with the opportunity to purchase aromatherapy products. Advice might include the use of a bath oil that will complement the treatment, or the use of an aromatic burner with appropriate oils. Oils can be given for the client to use as an inhalant by putting a few drops on a handkerchief. Other advice on lifestyle issues such as diet and exercise may be given to complement the aromatherapy treatments.

When the client returns for the next treatment, always discuss the effects of the previous treatment and be ready to adjust the oils and method of application to suit the client's needs.

Useful blends

The following blends are used as 7 drops to 15 ml of carrier oil (2 % solution).

To help sleep

- 4 drops of lavender, 2 drops of Roman chamomile, 1 drop of clary sage.
- 4 drops of lavender, 2 drops of ylang ylang, 1 drop of Roman chamomile.
- 3 drops of sandalwood, 2 drops of juniper, 2 drops of cypress.

To ease stress

- 3 drops of sandalwood, 2 drops of clary sage, 2 drops of juniper.
- 3 drops of frankincense, 2 drops of vetiver, 2 drops of lavender.
- 3 drops of mandarin, 2 drops of bergamot, 2 drops of Moroccan chamomile.

To uplift when feeling tired

- 3 drops of bergamot, 2 drops of sandalwood, 2 drops of Roman chamomile.
- 3 drops of lemongrass, 2 drops of benzoin, 2 drops of sandalwood.
- 3 drops of rosemary, 3 drops of peppermint, 1 drop of geranium.

For aches and pains after exercise

- 3 drops of juniper, 2 drops of eucalyptus, 2 drops of Roman chamomile.
- 3 drops of ginger, 2 drops of black pepper, 2 drops of rosemary.
- 3 drops of lavender, 2 drops of German chamomile, 2 drops of lemongrass.

For coughs and colds

- 3 drops of rosemary, 2 drops of eucalyptus, 2 drops of tea tree.
- 3 drops of lavender, 2 drops of peppermint, 2 drops of thyme ct. linalol.
- 3 drops of pine, 2 drops of eucalyptus, 2 drops of marjoram.

ACTIVITY

Keep a record of the blends you use, the clients they were used on and the results of the treatment.

Progress Check

Try to answer the following questions.

1 What carrier oil would you select for an elderly client with dry skin?
2 Why is gamma linoleic acid a useful ingredient in carrier oils?
3 Select pairs of oils that would be suitable for use with clients who:
    a) have a very stressed lifestyle
    b) feel very lethargic
    c) have weight and cellulite problems
    d) tend to get stiff and sore after an activity such as gardening.

Further uses for essential oils

Essential oils can be used effectively in ways other than massage. They can be used in skin care by mixing them with a bland cream or adding them to a basic face mask. They can be used in compresses, in baths and be diffused into the atmosphere.

Compresses

Compresses can be hot or cold. For hot compresses, a few drops of oil can be added to a bowl of hot water and a cloth or flannel dipped in and wrung out. This can then be placed on the affected area. They are useful to place on the back, for instance, while the rest of the body is being massaged and are particularly useful for backache or arthritic joints.

A cold compress is prepared in the same way using chilled water and is suitable for the forehead if the client has a headache or on a sprained joint.

Diffusion

Oils can be diffused into the atmosphere in a number of way. The commonest method is to use a pottery burner which contains a night light candle. A few drops of oil are placed in warm water in the saucer-shaped bowl over the candle. The heat from the night light speeds up the evaporation of the oil into the atmosphere. There are also electrical versions of these burners available.

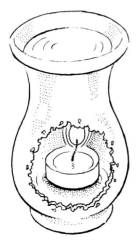

Figure 11.3 *Pottery oil burner*

A more effective way of spreading oils into the atmosphere is to use an electrically operated nebuliser or vapouriser which propels the oil into the air in a very fine mist.

Inhalation

A few drops of an essential oil can be placed in a bowl of hot water and the steam inhaled by the client using a towel over the head to prevent the steam escaping.

Drops of oil may be placed on a handkerchief or on some cotton wool which can be kept in a small container and be inhaled as necessary.

Home baths

Essential oils can be added directly to bath water just before getting in or can be mixed with a little carrier oil first. If added directly, the oil must be well mixed into the water before sitting in the bath to avoid letting the oils come into direct contact with the skin. If used with a carrier, the client must be careful not to slip.

Suggested oils for the bath:

- **for relaxing** – 6 drops of lavender with 4 of geranium; or 7 drops of Roman chamomile with 3 of basil
- **for colds** – 6 drops of pine with 6 of eucalyptus
- **for aches and pain**s – 4 drops of rosemary with 3 of Roman chamomile or juniper.

All these methods can be used to enhance and complement aromatherapy massage.

Key Terms

You need to know what these words mean. Go back through the chapter or check in the glossary to find out.

- Blend
- Carrier oils
- Compress
- Diffusion
- Inhalation
- Synergy
- Treatment plan

12 AROMATHERAPY MASSAGE

After working through this chapter you will be able to:
- prepare a client for aromatherapy massage
- adapt the principles of body massage to aromatherapy massage
- apply the principles of acupressure to body massage
- apply the principles of massage and acupressure to face and scalp massage
- give home advice to clients following aromatherapy massage
- explain how aromatherapy is being used in some medical settings.

Although essential oils can be used in many ways, massage is the most important and commonly used method of applying them in aromatherapy. This is because massage combines the therapeutic power of touch with the properties of the oils. Massage provides a very effective way of introducing the oils into the body. As the skin absorbs the oils, a useful amount will be taken into the bloodstream in the relatively short time that a body massage takes.

In general, the conditions and legislation that cover the practice of aromatherapy will be the same as those covering the practice of massage and are described in chapter 1.

The effects of aromatherapy massage will consist of:
- the effects of the massage
- the effects of the oils used.

aromatherapy oils can be administered to the body using a typical body massage routine and different aromatherapists will have quite different techniques depending on their training and experience. However, in general, the massage used in aromatherapy treatments is a relaxing massage using mainly effleurage and stroking movements and omitting the percussion and more vigorous petrissage movements. Instead of these, many therapists integrate finger pressures into their massage which may be called acupressure or shiatsu pressures or neuro-muscular techniques.

SAFE PRACTICE

Contraindications to aromatherapy massage will consist of:
- contraindications to massage
- contraindications to the oils to be used
- contraindications to acupressure.

Acupressure

This refers to many treatment systems that manipulate the acupuncture points on the body by pressure rather than by needles as is the case with acupuncture. The acu points are found along twelve pairs of meridians or channels which pass down the body. It is said that energies flow along these meridians which govern the body's systems (see Figure 8.3, page 146, chapter 8).

When pressure is applied to a point on a meridian, it stimulates local nerves and tissues and also influences the flow of energy through that and other meridians. The basic philosophy of acu points comes from traditional Chinese systems of healing, however most Eastern societies will have pressures in their massage therapies. Similar pressures are found in Japanese shiatsu and Indian head massage as well in reflexology treatments to the feet.

All of these techniques are part of a whole philosophy of treatment attempting to return the energy or chi of the body to a state where Yin (negative) and Yang (positive) qualities are in balance.

Acupressure treatment is very different from the usual Swedish-style massage, as there are no smooth flowing strokes, just pressure and stretching. However, some pressures applied with the fingers or the thumb can be integrated into a Western-style massage very successfully and more can be used as a knowledge of the meridian lines is gained. Sliding pressures applied with the thumb or the hand along meridians are particularly useful in aromatherapy as oils are always used.

Pressures

When using pressure techniques, the thumbs are the usual tools for applying pressure as the acu points are mostly placed in thumb-sized hollows. In some areas, a finger may be used often supported by the adjacent finger. The heel of the hand may be used over larger areas such as the side of the buttocks.

Pressure should be applied in a firm, controlled manner with body weight controlling the amount of pressure. No poking or roughness should be used and pressure should be moderate to light. When sliding pressure is applied, it should be even and the sliding movement steady, with care being taken not to cause discomfort by pulling on hair or skin.

The client should breathe out when pressure is applied to the back or chest and breath in between pressures.

Pressures are usually performed only once over the area, whereas the traditional massage movements will be repeated a number of times depending on the time available and the speed of the strokes.

REMEMBER
Use your hands and eyes to check the client's responses.

SAFE PRACTICE

Contraindications to pressures are the same as those for massage – don't press over any tender or fragile area and, if pain occurs, use very light pressure. Take care that nails do not dig in.

Routine for an aromatherapy treatment

◆ Consultation – which should take at least half an hour in the first instance.
◆ Complete a consultation card.

- Obtain the client's signature.
- Check for contraindications to massage and oils.
- Select appropriate oils and check their acceptability with the client.
- Mix the oils and check their acceptability with client – mix enough 2 % mixture for the body and 1% mixture for the face.
- Check that all necessary oils, creams, towels, cotton wool and tissues are close to hand.
- Suggest the client empties their bladder.
- An infrared treatment may be given to warm the client but saunas and steam baths are not suitable.
- The client lies supine, warm and well-covered by towels.
- Cover the hair with a light, loose cloth or towel unless the scalp is to be included.
- If the scalp is to be included, ask the client if oil may be used on the hair.
- Deep cleanse the face if facial massage is to be included.
- Place a little of the 1 % oil mixture on the client's hands and ask them to inhale and lightly stroke the cheeks with the oil mixture. If there is only 2 % mixture available apply a little to the client's upper lip.

REMEMBER
During treatment only the part to be worked on should be uncovered.

SAFE PRACTICE

Always take care to avoid getting oils in the eyes or on the eyelids.

The order and timing of massage for an aromatherapy treatment can be adapted from the usual full body massage routine found in chapter 6.

Suggested order and approximate timing for a full body aromatherapy massage including face and scalp

Total time taken: one and a half hours.

The client turns to lie prone with the hands under the forehead or by the sides.

1 Back, which presents the largest area for the oils to absorbed quickly – 20 minutes.
2 Back of left leg and buttock – 5 minutes.
3 Back of right leg and buttock – 5 minutes.

The client turns over to lie on the back (with a pillow under the head if necessary).

4 Front of left leg and foot – 10 minutes.
5 Front of right leg and foot – 10 minutes.
6 Abdomen – 5 minutes.
7 Right arm – 5 minutes.
8 Left arm – 5 minutes.
9 Scalp – 5 minutes.
10 Face and shoulders – 20 minutes.

The routine can be adapted to suit the client and therapist. In this routine, the back is treated first to allow for maximum absorption of the oils, but equally the face and scalp could be treated first.

Suggested routine for the back
Expose the whole length of the back from shoulders to buttocks. (Only those movements not described in chaper 6 are explained in detail.)

1 Full back stretch (once only)
Stance Walk- or stride-standing facing across the client.

Hands With arms straight at the elbow, one hand is placed on the upper back, the other on the upper part of the sacrum with the arms crossed. Apply stretch to the whole length of the spine taking care not to press the face down into the couch.

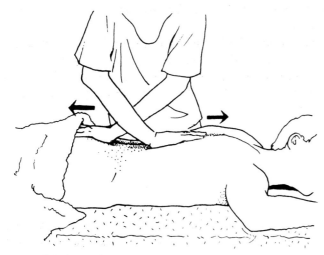

Figure 12.1 *Full back stretch*

2 Pressures to the base of the skull (once only)
Stance Walk-standing facing the head.

Hands One hand supports the head while pressure is applied with the other.

Support the head with the left hand, apply pressures with the right thumb on the left side of the head against the base of the skull from the outside to the centre finishing with a pressure at the centre. Repeat pressures with the middle finger of the right hand on the right side of the head.

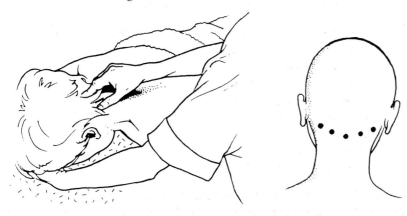

Figure 12.2 *Pressures to the base of the skull*

3 Apply oil to the back

Take about a third of the total oil mixed for a body massage and apply it to the back with sweeping effleurage movements.

4 Reverse effleurage

See page 117, chapter 6.

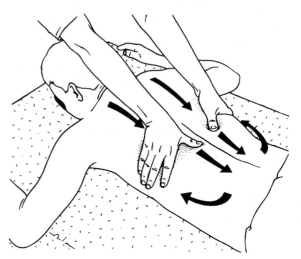

Figure 12.3 *Reverse effleurage*

5 T-shaped effleurage

See page 118, chapter 6.

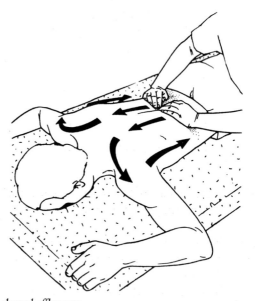

Figure 12.4 *T-shaped effleurage*

6 Circular stroking around the scapulae

See page 118, chapter 6.

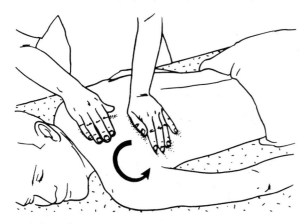

Figure 12.5 *Circular stroking around the scapulae*

7 Figure-of-eight around the scapulae

See page 119, chapter 6.

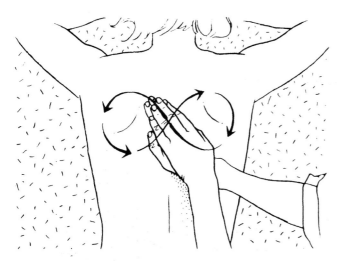

Figure 12.6 *Figure of eight stroking around the scapulae*

8 Pressures down one side of the spine (once only)

Stance Walk- or stride-standing facing across the client.

Hands With fingertips resting lightly on the back at shoulder level, place the thumbs together and facing each other. The thumbs should be in the hollow between the spine and the erector spinae muscles of the back. Press down firmly but gently, asking the client to breathe out as you press. Maintain the pressure for a count of about 4 to 5 (can be quicker if the client requires stimulating rather than relaxation), and release moving down a little way while the client breathes in. Pressures are applied in this way all the way down one side of the spine. The thumbs should fall naturally into the hollows between vertebrae.

REMEMBER
Make sure your nails don't dig in.

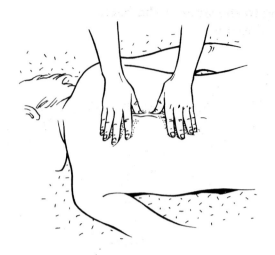

Figure 12.7 *Pressures down the side of spine*

9 Sliding pressures down the same side (once only)

Stance   As for movement 8.

Hands   In same position as for 8.

Apply steady pressure with both thumbs and keeping the pressure constant throughout, slide the lower thumb down an inch and push the other to meet it. When the level of the sacrum is reached lift the thumbs and slide the fingers up to shoulder level to repeat pressures and sliding on the other side

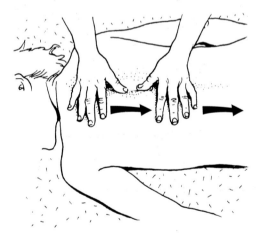

Figure 12.8 *Sliding pressures down the side of the spine*

10 Pressures down other side of spine (once only)
Repeat movement 8.

11 Sliding pressures down the other side of spine (once only)
Repeat movement 9.

12 Wringing to the sides of the back
See page 122, chapter 6.

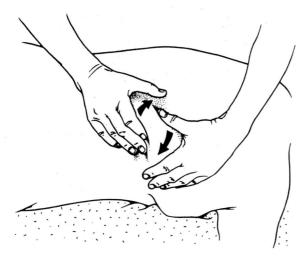

Figure 12.9 *Wringing to the sides of the back*

13 Skin rolling to the sides of the back
See page 122, chapter 6.

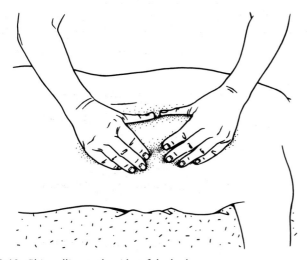

Figure 12.10 *Skin rolling to the sides of the back*

14 Effleurage towards the lymph nodes (lower cervical, axillary and inguinal)
See page 121, chapter 6.

15 Transverse stroking to the lumbar region
See page 122, chapter 6.

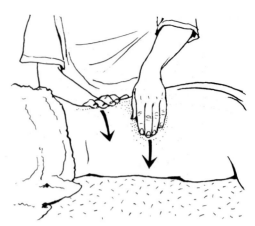

Figure 12.11 *Transverse stroking to the lumbar region*

16 Circular thumb kneading over the sacrum and iliac region

Stance Walk-standing facing up the body.

Hands Resting lightly at waist level with the thumbs on either side of the spine.

Pressure is applied with the thumbs which move in small circles outwards along the top of the iliac crest and down the sides of the hips. Return thumbs to the centre about an inch lower down and repeat the circular movements. Repeat twice so that four rows of kneadings are completed.

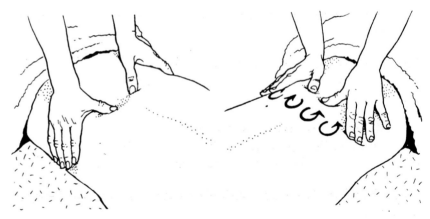

Figure 12.12 *Circular thumb kneading over the sacrum and iliac region*

Complete this movement by applying pressure with the fingers or heel of the hand to the sides of the buttocks, hold for a moment then release.

17 Effleurage to the sides of the back with alternate hands

Stance Walk-standing facing up the body.

Hands One hand starts at the base of the spine pushing upwards and outwards to the side of the body. The other hand then starts the same movement a little higher up so that one hand is always in contact until the whole side is covered. Repeat on the other side.

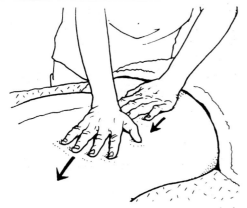

Figure 12.13 *Effleurage to the side of the back with alternate hands*

18 T-shaped effleurage
Cover the back with towels tucking them in over the shoulders. See page 118, chapter 6.

Progress Check

Practise this back routine until it can be performed fluently in 20 minutes.

Legs

About a third of the remaining body oil should be used for the backs of both legs.

Suggested routine for the back of the leg
(Only those movements not described in chapter 6 are explained in detail.)

1 Apply oil to the backs of the legs
Apply oil with effleurage to the whole length of both legs including the feet and buttocks and cover the leg not being treated first.

2 Flat handed effleurage with alternate hands to the length of the leg

Stance   Stride-standing facing across the client.

Hands   One hand is placed on the leg at ankle level, the other at knee level. Both are placed with the hands firmly cupped over the leg so that pressure is applied through the palms not the fingers.

Move both hands slowly and steadily up the leg keeping the same distance between them and the pressure firm and steady. When the lower hand reaches the knee, it is removed but not before the upper hand reaches the top of the thigh and is brought down to ankle level. This hand now moves firmly up as far as the knee and then the free hand starts at the ankle again and they both continue together. Repeat this a number of times always with one or both hands in contact.

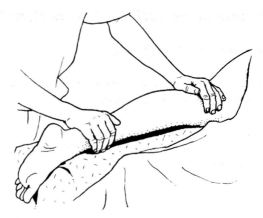

Figure 12.14 *Flat-handed effleurage with alternate hands to length of leg*

3 Wringing to the thigh and buttock
See page 112, chapter 6.

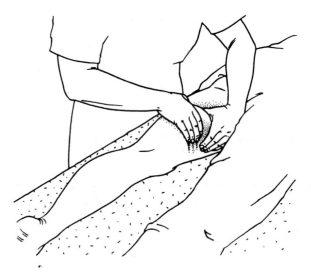

Figure 12.15 *Wringing to the back of the leg and thigh*

4 Effleurage to the thigh and buttock
See page 111, chapter 6.

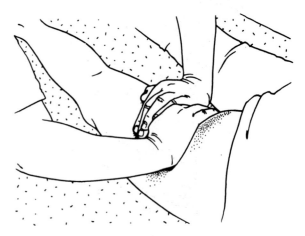

Figure 12.16 *Effleurage to the thigh and buttock*

5 Sliding pressure to the midline of the thigh with alternate hands

Stance   Walk-standing facing up the body.

Hands   One hand rests on the midline of the thigh just above the knee with fingers pointing up the thigh.

Applying firm and quite deep pressure, slide the hand slowly up the thigh to the base of the buttock. Before lifting it off, start the same movement with the other hand.

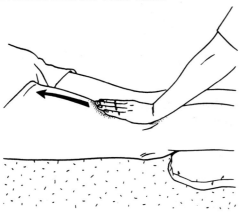

Figure 12.17 *Sliding pressure to the midline of the thigh*

6 Effleurage to the whole back of the leg
See page 224, chapter 6.

7 Single-handed effleurage to the calf with the knee bent

Stance   Walk-standing at ankle level facing up the couch.

Hands   With one hand under the ankle, lift the lower leg so that the knee is bent almost at right angles.

Place the other hand so that it is cupped over the calf just above the ankle and applying pressure with the palm, stroke firmly down to the knee. Repeat a number of times and place the lower leg down gently.

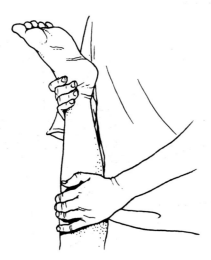

Figure 12.18 *Single-handed effleurage to the calf with the knee bent*

8 Sliding pressures with thumbs from the ankle to the knee

Stance   Stand at the end of the couch.

Hands   Cup the sides of the ankle with thumbs lying close and parallel on top of the leg.

Keeping thumb tips together and applying pressure evenly with the length of the thumbs and the palms of the hands, slide the hands up to the knee. Release the pressure to return the hands to ankle level to repeat. This movement should leave a 'stocking seam' line in the oil.

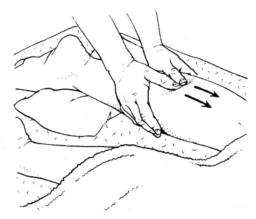

Figure 12.19 *Sliding pressures with thumbs from the ankle to the knee*

9 Effleurage to the whole back of the leg

Repeat movement 6.

Repeat movements 1–9 on the back of the other leg. Ask the client to turn over for the massage to the front of the leg and place pillows for support where necessary.

Suggested routine for the front of the leg

(Only those movements not described in chapter 6 are explained in detail.)

Spread the oil with firm sweeping effleurage to both legs including the feet, using about one third of the remaining oil.

Cover one leg with a towel.

1 Effleurage to the sides and front of the whole leg

See page 84, chapter 6.

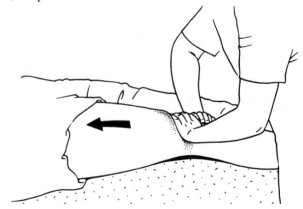

Figure 12.20 *Effleurage to the sides and front of the leg*

2 *Effleurage to the thigh*
See page 85, chapter 6.

3 Double-handed kneading to the thigh
See page 85, chapter 6.

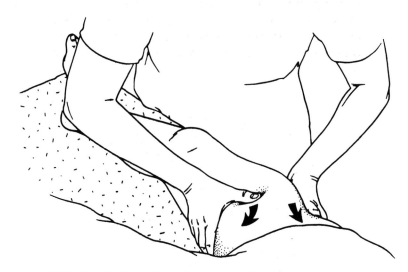

Figure 12.21 *Double-handed kneading to the thigh*

4 Wringing to the thigh muscles
See page 86, chapter 6.

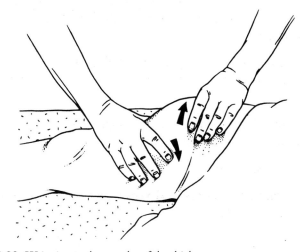

Figure 12.22 *Wringing to the muscles of the thigh*

5 Stroking around the knee
See page 87, chapter 6.

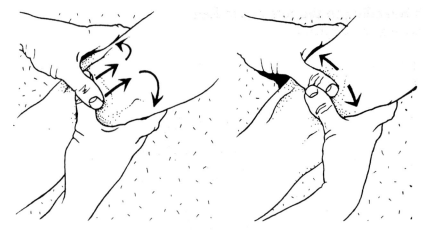

Figure 12.23 *Stroking around the knees*

6 Effleurage to the foot and lower leg

Stance   Walk-standing at end of couch.

Hands   One on top of the foot and one under the foot.

Effleurage up the sides of the calf to the knee, returning with the pads of the thumbs applying gentle pressure to the tibialis muscle at the front of the leg.

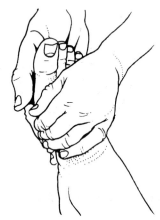

Figure 12.24 *Effleurage to the foot*

7 Effleurage to the foot
See page 90, chapter 6.

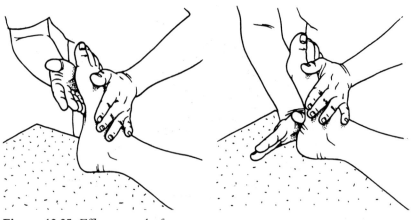

Figure 12.25 *Effleurage to the foot*

8 Kneading to the sole of the foot

See page 90, chapter 6.

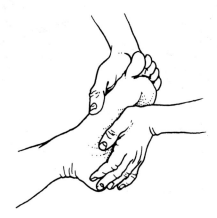

Figure 12.26 *Kneading to the sole of the foot*

9 Thumb stroking to the top of the foot

See page 90, chapter 6.

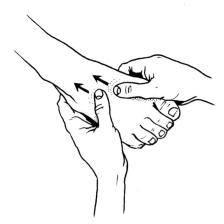

Figure 12.27 *Thumb stroking to the top of the foot*

10 Thumb stroking across the sole of the foot

See page 91, chapter 6.

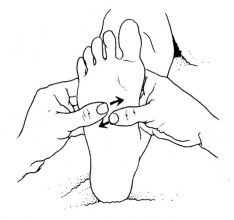

Figure 12.28 *Thumb stroking across the sole of the foot*

11 Kneading to the toes
See page 92, chapter 6.

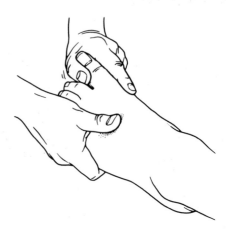

Figure 12.29 *Kneading to the toes*

12 Repeat effleurage to the whole front leg
Repeat movement 1.

Repeat movements 1–12 on other leg.

Abdomen

Suggested routine for the abdomen
(Only those movements not described in chapter 6 are explained in detail.)

Fold the towels back to expose the abdomen. Place a small rolled-up towel under the knees to relax the abdomen. Take a third of the remaining oil and spread with clockwise circular strokes.

1 Effleurage to the front and sides of the abdomen
See pages 107 and 108, chapter 6.

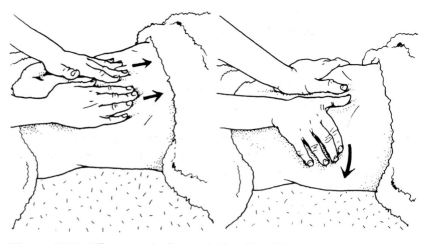

Figure 12.30 *Effleurage to the front and sides of the abdomen*

2 Circular stroking in a clockwise direction with alternate hands

See pages 107 and 108, chapter 6.

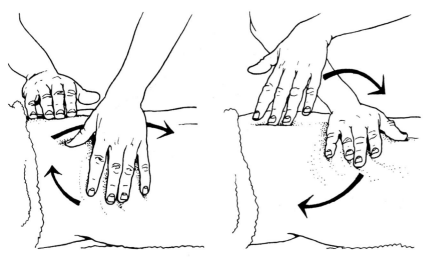

Figure 12.31 *Circular stroking in a clockwise direction with alternate hands*

3 Circular kneading over the colon

See page 108, chapter 6.

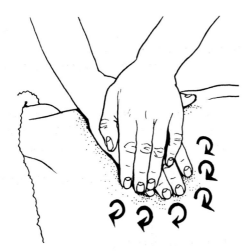

Figure 12.32 *Circular kneading over the colon*

4 Stroking to the sides of the waist with alternate hands

Stance   Walk-standing at waist level facing up the couch.

Hands   One hand placed on the lower ribs strokes downwards and in to the centre followed by the other hand a little lower down. Use alternate hands to cover the side from ribs to hips. Repeat on the other side.

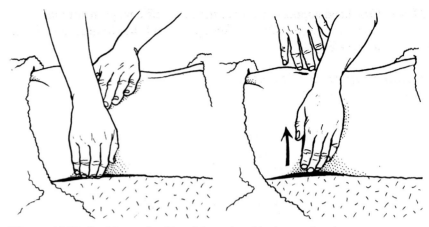

Figure 12.33 *Stroking to the sides of the waist with alternate hands*

5 Effleurage to the front and sides of the abdomen
See page 109, chapter 6.

Arms

Suggested routine for the arms
Apply the remaining body oil to both arms using sweeping effleurage strokes. Support the arm fully during the massage.

1 Effleurage to the front of the arm
See page 95, chapter 6.

2 Effleurage to the back of the arm including the shoulder
See page 95, chapter 6.

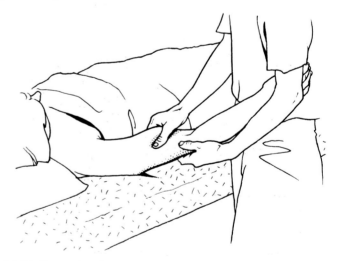

Figure 12.34 *Supporting the arm*

3 Effleurage from the elbow to the shoulder
Stance   Walk-standing at waist level. The client places a hand on the chest with elbow at right angles.

Hands One hand supports the arm, the other effleurages from the elbow to the shoulder and sweeps around the shoulder and down to the elbow.

4 Effleurage to the forearm
See page 97, chapter 6.

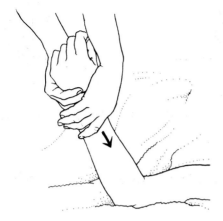

Figure 12.35 *Effleurage to the forearm*

5 Sliding pressure up the midline of the forearm
Stance Walk-standing facing along the arm which should be supported.

Hands One hand supports the forearm, the other rests at the front of the wrist with the fingers pointing to the elbow.

Slide the hand with firm pressure up the centre of the forearm to the elbow and lightly return.

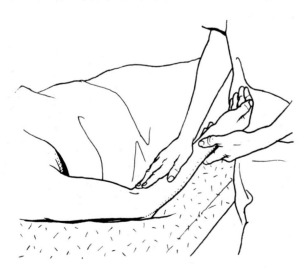

Figure 12.36 *Sliding pressure up the midline of the forearm*

6 Thumb stroking to the palm of the hand
See page 98, chapter 6.

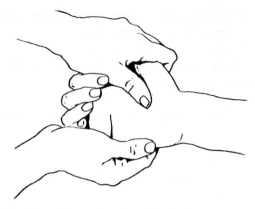

Figure 12.37 *Thumb stroking to the palm of the hand*

7 Thumb stroking to the back of the hand
See page 100, chapter 6.

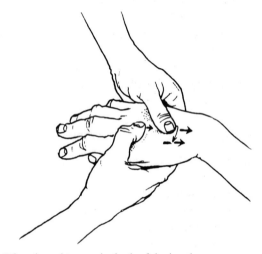

Figure 12.38 *Thumb stroking to the back of the hand*

8 Effleurage to the whole arm
Repeat movements 1–2.

Repeat movements 1–8 on the other arm.

This concludes the body massage.

Summary of movements

Back

1 Full back stretch.
2 Pressures to the base of the skull.
3 Apply oil to the whole surface of the back – about a third of the total body oil can be used.
4 Reverse effleurage, shoulders to hips.
5 T-shaped effleurage, hips to shoulders.
6 Circular stroking around the left and right scapulae.

7   Figure-of-eight reinforced stroking around the scapulae.
8   Pressures down one side of the spine.
9   Sliding pressures down same side of the spine.
10 & 11   Repeat of 8 and 9 on the other side of the spine.
12   Wringing to the sides of the back.
13   Skin rolling to the sides of the back.
14   Effleurage towards the lymph nodes (lower cervical, axillary and inguinal).
15   Transverse stroking to the lumbar region.
16   Circular thumb kneading over the sacrum and iliac region.
17   Effleurage to the sides of the back with alternate hands.
18   T-shaped effleurage.

Back of the leg

1   Apply the oil with sweeping effleurage strokes to include the foot and buttock.
2   Flat-handed effleurage with alternate hands to the whole leg.
3   Wringing to the thigh and buttock.
4   Effleurage to the thigh and buttock.
5   Sliding pressure to the midline of the thigh with alternate hands.
6   Effleurage to the whole leg.
7   Single-handed effleurage to the calf with the knee bent.
8   Sliding pressures with thumbs from ankle to knee.
9   Effleurage to the whole leg.

Front of the leg

1   Effleurage to the sides and front of the whole leg including the foot.
2   Effleurage to the thigh.
3   Double-handed kneading to the thigh.
4   Wringing to the thigh muscles.
5   Stroking around the knee.
6   Effleurage to the foot and lower leg.
7   Effleurage to the foot.
8   Kneading to the sole of the foot.
9   Thumb stroking to the top of the foot.
10   Thumb stroking across the sole of the foot.
11   Kneading to the toes.
12   Effleurage to the whole leg.

Abdomen

1   Effleurage to the front and sides of the abdomen.
2   Circular stroking in a clockwise direction with alternate hands.
3   Circular kneading over the colon.
4   Stroking to the sides of the waist with alternate hands.
5   Effleurage to the front and sides of the abdomen.

Arm

1   Effleurage to the front of the arm.
2   Effleurage to the back of the arm.
3   Effleurage from elbow to shoulder.
4   Effleurage to the forearm.
5   Sliding pressure up the midline of the forearm.

6 Thumb stroking to the palm of the hand.
7 Thumb stroking to the back of the hand.
8 Effleurage to the whole hand.

Once the whole body massage is complete, cover the client, check for comfort and warmth and proceed with the facial and scalp massage using the 1 % mixture for the face.

Facial and scalp massage

If the scalp as well as the face and chest is to be treated then approximately 10 ml of carrier oil with 2–3 drops of essential oils will be needed. 5 ml will be adequate if only the face and chest are to be treated.

If the client prefers, the scalp can be massaged with dry hands followed by the facial massage with aromatherapy oils.

The therapist can sit at the head of the couch for part of this massage.

Scalp

Place a little oil in the palm of one hand and dabble the fingertips of the other in it.

1 Apply oil to the scalp
Apply oil to the scalp with the fingertips using small circular movements to cover the whole scalp.

2 Pressures to the midline
With one thumb resting on the other apply pressure at the midline of the hairline, release the pressure and repeat gradually moving backwards to the crown of the head.

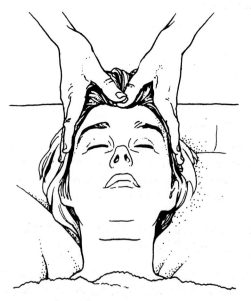

Figure 12.39 *Pressures to the midline*

3 Repeat of pressures

Repeat the pressures described in movement 2 a half inch to either side of the centre with thumbs from hairline to crown and continue working outwards to temples.

4 Friction to the scalp

With fingertips clawed along the hairline, move them in deep slow circular movements so that the scalp moves over the bone. Gradually work backwards altering the position of the hands so that the whole head is covered.

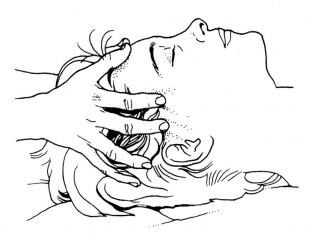

Figure 12.40 *Friction to the scalp*

5 Stroke the fingertips through the hair from the hairline to the ends of the hair

Techniques used in Indian head massage may also be used (see chapter 8).

Face

Any appropriate facial massage routine may be used so long as the neck and chest are included.

GOOD PRACTICE

The therapist should wash or wipe the hands before beginning to treat the face.

Suggested facial routine
1 Apply oil to the face

Apply oil with circular movements over the whole face and neck. Start with the neck, chest, shoulders, cheeks, sides of nose and forehead. Avoid the eyelids with aromatherapy oils. Finish with gentle pressure applied with the palms of the hands to both temples.

REMEMBER
A 1% solution is used on the face.

2 Effleurage to the chest, shoulders and neck

Stance Standing at head of couch.

Hands Lying flat on the chest, hands pass out to shoulders, around the point of the shoulder and up the back of the neck with a slight pull on the base of the skull.

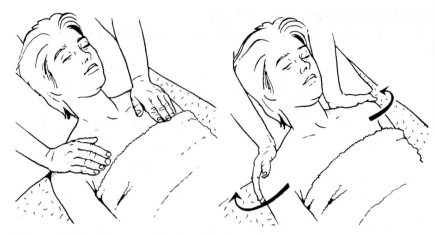

Figure 12.41 *Effleurage to the chest, shoulders and neck*

3 Finger kneading to the upper back

Hands Fingers under the shoulder apply kneading to the trapezius muscles.

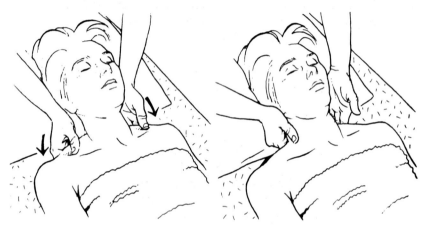

Figure 12.42 *Finger kneading to the upper back*

4 Effleurage to the neck

Hands Alternate hands stroke upwards on the neck from the shoulders and chest to the jawline to cover the whole neck.

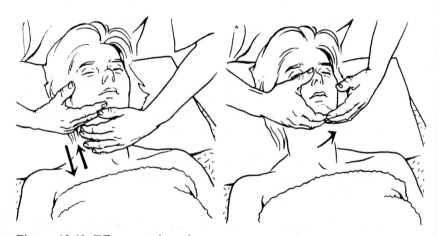

Figure 12.43 *Effleurage to the neck*

5 Effleurage from chin to cheek

Hands Fingers linked under the chin stroke upwards to the cheeks.

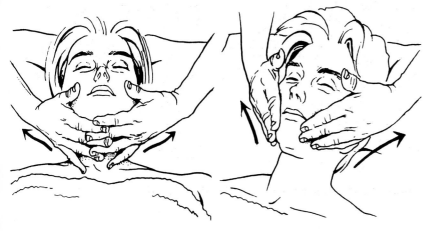

Figure 12.44 *Chin to cheek effleurage*

6 Finger pressures on the cheekbones

Hands Place the thumbs on the forehead and the index and middle fingers on the sides of the nose. Apply pressures with the fingers along the top of the cheekbone to the temples.

Repeat lower down along the cheekbones and again along the lower edge of the cheekbones.

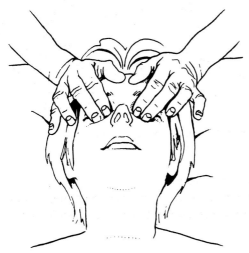

Figure 12.45 *Finger pressures on the cheekbones*

7 Circular finger stroking

Hands With the middle fingers starting at the sides of the nostril, stroke up the sides of the nose to the bridge of the nose, along the top of the eyebrows down to the cheekbone and in to the sides of the nostrils again. Both fingers should move at the same time.

8 Pressures to the eyebrows and forehead

Hands Fingers resting on the temples and thumbs together between eyebrows.

Apply pressures along the length of the eyebrows then repeat an inch higher and again until the whole forehead is covered.

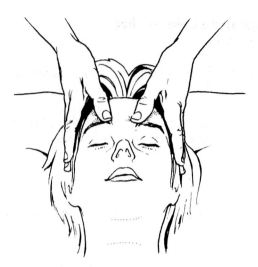

Figure 12.46 *Pressures to the eyebrows*

9 Stroking across the forehead

Hands With fingers resting on the temples and the base of the thumbs resting on the centre of the forehead, stroke outwards with the thumbs to meet the fingers.

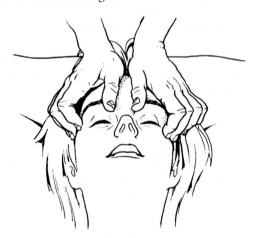

Figure 12.47 *Stroking across the forehead*

10 Alternate hand stroking to the forehead

Hands With alternate palms stroke upwards from the temple to the hairline across the forehead to the other temple.

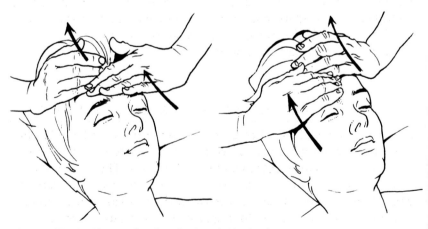

Figure 12.48 *Alternate hand stroking to the forehead*

11 Effleurage from chin to cheek

Repeat movement 5.

12 Effleurage to the chest, shoulders and neck

Repeat movement 2.

This completes the treatment and after allowing a little time, the head of the couch can be raised to allow the client to get up.

REMEMBER

As the massage comes to an end, make the movements slower and lighter.

Progress Check

Practise the facial and scalp routine until you are able to perform it fluently.

A whole body massage may not be required or appropriate. Individual parts of the body may be treated by aromatherapy massage taking less time and costing a proportional amount. For example:

- back massage – 30 minutes
- feet and lower legs – 15 minutes each leg
- face and scalp – 30 minutes
- face, chest and shoulders – 30 minutes.

If only a small part of the body is to be treated, the essential oils used may be used in slightly stronger concentrations. 3 % to 4 % may be used on the body but not the face and only if the safety of the oil has been checked.

ACTIVITY

Consider what types of client would benefit most from an aromatherapy massage consisting of:

a) full body
b) feet and lower legs
c) face and scalp
d) face, chest and shoulders.

Following a body massage, a client should be advised to leave the oils on the body for a few hours in order to maximise the effects. It is also wise to tell the client whether the oils used could have a sedative or stimulating effect, especially if the client is driving.

Massage and aromatherapy in a medical setting

The growth in popularity of complementary therapies is reflected in the number of health care professionals showing an interest in training and in using these therapies in the treatment of patients. There is a real desire among nurses, physiotherapists and occupational therapists to return to their caring role rather than the medical model that has been the trend for many years. The term 'holistic approach' is being used more and more where all aspects of the individual being treated are considered rather than just the physical. Non-medical personnel who are fully trained in complementary therapies are also being welcomed into hospitals, hospices and other care units to work together with more orthodox therapists for the benefit of the patients. For example, a major London teaching hospital employs three aromatherapists in the oncology (cancer) department, giving aromatherapy treatments to patients to help in their palliative care. This development is being repeated in many National Health and private centres of care especially in the care of the elderly, mentally ill, terminally ill and multi-handicapped.

The following are some examples of the way in which massage and aromatherapy are being used.

Working with the elderly
Aromatherapy has a clear role to play in the care of the elderly and in helping those with age-related conditions. Many conditions are treated by nurses who are also qualified aromatherapists.

- For respiratory conditions where the immune system is depressed, diffusers can be used to disperse oils into the atmosphere to inhibit the spread of bacterial infections.
- Poor circulation is quite common and elderly patients may benefit from warm aromatherapy footbaths using such oils as marjoram, black pepper or ginger as well as aromatherapy massage.
- Footbaths might also be used to help patients with fungal infections of the feet when lemon, cypress or tea tree might be used.
- The psychological effects are important too, especially with confused patients. Aromas can stimulate memories and encourage patients to talk about themselves. These pleasant aromas, combined with the therapeutic benefits of gentle touch and massage, can stimulate the patients to take more interest in their surroundings.
- Sleep patterns can be influenced. A trial to evaluate the effects of lavender diffusion on the sleep patterns of patients with dementia was carried out in 1993. The trial ran over a 7-week period, in a hospital, using an electric diffuser. The results showed a significant improvement in the sleep patterns of the patients.
- Physiotherapists in Scotland, working with the elderly mentally frail, used aromatherapy massage to replace splinting which was being used to prevent flexion deformities of the hands. The splinting was necessary to prevent the hands becoming fixed in a clenched fist. It was found that if nurses and physiotherapists massaged the hands with relaxing blends of oils for a few minutes in each hour and the hands left lying loosely over a rolled towel, then the splinting could be dispensed with.

Labour ward
Midwives at the John Radcliffe Maternity Hospital in Oxford, wanting to find a way of relieving pain and calming women in labour set out to evaluate the use of essential oils for the purpose. The project lasted 6 months and the oils used were lavender, clary sage, peppermint, eucalyptus, chamomile, frankincense, jasmine, rose, lemon and mandarin.

The oils were used in baths, footbaths, inhaled or massaged. The most effective oil used was lavender with peppermint and clary sage also showing good results. There was a high degree of satisfaction from the women and the midwives and the use of essential oils has been retained in the labour ward.

Intensive care
Research in the intensive and coronary care unit of the Royal Sussex County Hospital showed that massage and the use of essential oils reduced the heart rate and breathing rate in most of the patients tested and seemed to be more effective than massage alone.

The feet were massaged with lavender in a carrier oil and comparison was made with patients who were massaged with carrier oil alone. The drop in the heart rate was significantly greater in the lavender group.

Anxiety
Trials at Birmingham Women's hospital have been carried out with the aim of finding out whether massage or inhalation with essential oils could help reduce blood pressure in patients before surgery. Anxiety can increase blood pressure, which may lead to cancellation of the surgery or an increase in drugs needed. Aromatherapy has shown a good success rate so far.

Children
Aromatherapy and massage are currently being used by many occupational therapists in a variety of settings to develop relationships, relieve anxiety and to help physical function.

One example is where the occupational therapist massaged the hands of children using lavender oil to relax and mobilise the hands before exercise. Other uses may be to diffuse the essential oils into the atmosphere to promote concentration or relaxation.

Children with multi-handicaps such as those whose sight and hearing is impaired have been shown to benefit from use of essential oils with gentle massage, particularly in building relationships with therapists and teachers.

Alcoholism
Work is being carried on in a centre for women with alcoholism who are trying to control their drinking. Treatment is initially aimed at comforting and nurturing the women emotionally, using oils such as rose and lavender. Later, physical problems such as muscular tension and a depressed immune system are addressed. It has been found that benefits include an improved self-image, reduced emotional stress and alleviation of some of the physical problems associated with alcoholism.

Constipation
Children and adults in residential care often suffer from constipation. Treatment by aromatherapy massage to the abdomen has been found to be a good alternative to the use of enemas. It is much less intrusive a treatment and much less likely to cause discomfort to the patient.

Care settings
There are many more instances of the use of aromatherapy and other complementary therapies in hospitals, hospices and other care settings. With the acceptance of the value of such treatments by medical

professionals in future there will be an increasing need for qualified aromatherapists and for medical personnel to become qualified.

ACTIVITY

Try to carry out a literature search in professional journals and collect references to the use of massage and aromatherapy in a variety of medical settings.

Key Terms

You need to know what these words mean. Go back through the chapter or check in the glossary to find out.

- Acupressure
- Diffusion
- Psychological effects
- Therapeutic
- Palliative

BIBLIOGRAPHY AND FURTHER READING

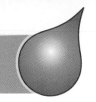

Barclay, J., 'The Story of Care in Our Hands', *Physiotherapy*, May 1994 vol. 80 no. 5.

Beck, M. *The Theory and Practice of Therapeutic Massage,* Milady Publishing Company, 1988.

Brown, Denise, *Aromatherapy,* Headway Lifeguides Series, 1993.

Burns, E. and Blamey, C., 'Soothing Scents in Childbirth', *The International Journal of Aromatherapy*, 1994 vol. 4 no. 1.

Corbett, M., 'The Use and Abuse of Massage and Exercise', *The Practitioner*, Jan 1972 vol. 208.

Cowmeadow, O., *The Art of Shiatsu,* Element Books Ltd, 1992.

Davis, P. *Aromatherapy, an A–Z,* C.W. Daniel Company Ltd, 1990.

Ernst, E. et al., 'Massages Cause Changes in Blood Fluidity', *Physiotherapy*, 1987 vol. 73 no. 1.

Fire, M., 'Providing Massage Therapy in a Psychiatric Hospital', *International Journal of Alternative and Complementary Medicine*, June 1994.

Gillam, L., 'Lymphoedema and Physiotherapists: Control not Cure', *Physiotherapy*, December 1994 vol. 80 no.12.

Grisogono, V., *Sports Injuries,* Churchill Livingstone, 1989.

Hayward, L., *Indian Head Massage*, Conservatree, 1997.

Henry, J. et al., 'Lavender for Night Sedation of People with Dementia', *International Journal of Aromatherapy*, 1994 vol. 6 no. 2.

Herring, M., 'Aromatherapy – Making Connections', *International Journal of Aromatherapy*, 1994 vol. 6 no. 1.

Hollis, M., *Massage for Therapists*, Blackwell Scientific Publications, 1987.

Hovind, H. and Nielsen, S., 'Effect of massage on Blood Flow in Skeletal Muscle', *Scandinavian Journal of Rehabilitation Medicine*, Med 6: 74–77, 1974.

Holey, E. and Cook, E., *Therapeutic Massage*, WB Saunders Company Ltd, 1998.

International School of Aromatherapy, *A Safety Guide on the Use of Essential Oils*, Nature by Nature Oils Ltd, London, 1993.

Lawless, Julia, *The Encyclopaedia of Essential Oils*, Element Books Ltd, 1992.

Lidell, L., Thomas, S., Beresford Cooke, C., Porter, A., *The Book of Massage*, Ebury Press, 1987.

Liechti, E., *Shiatsu, Japanese Massage for Health and Fitness*, Element Books, 1992.

Lavabre, M., *Aromatherapy Workbook*, Healing Arts Press USA, 1990.

Lundberg, P., *The Book of Shiatsu*, Gaia Books Ltd, 1992.

Marshall Cavendish, *How the Body Works*, Marshall Cavendish,1979.

Maxwell Hudson, C., *The Complete Book of Massage*, Dorling Kindersley, 1988.

Minett, P., Wayne, D., Rubenstein, D., *Human Form and Function*, Collins International, 1992.

Pitman, V., MacKenzie, K., *Reflexology: A Practical Approach*, Stanley Thornes (Publishers) Ltd, 1997.

Price L., *Carrier Oils for Aromatherapy and Massage*, Riverhead, 1999.

Price, S., *Practical Aromatherapy*, Thorsons Publishing Group, 1987.

Price, S., and Price, L., *Aromatherapy for Health Professionals,* Churchill Livingstone, 1995.

Quinter, J., 'Apropos Rub, Rub, Rubbish, Massage in the Ninteenth Century', *Physiotherapy*, 1993 vol. 79 no. 1.

Roberts, P., 'Theoretical Models of Physiotherapy', *Physiotherapy*, June 1994 vol. 80 no. 6.

Sanderson, H., Ruddle, J., 'Aromatherapy and Occupational Therapy', *British Journal of Occupational Therapy*, 1992, 55(8).

Sachs, M., *Ayurvedic Beauty Care*, Lotus Press, 1994.

Simms, J., *A Practical Guide to Beauty Therapy*, 2nd edition, Stanley Thornes (Publishers) Ltd, 1998.

Sigerist, H.E., *A History of Medicine*, Oxford University Press Inc., 1951.

Tisserand, R., 'Aromatherapy Today', *International Journal of Aromatherapy*, 1993 vol. 5 no. 4.

Tortora, G. and Grabowski, S.R., *Principles of Anatomy and Physiology*, John Wiley & Sons Inc., 2000.

Vickers, A., *Massage and Aromatherapy*, Stanley Thornes (Publishers) Ltd, 1996.

Woolfson, A. and Hewitt, D., 'Intensive Aroma Care', *International Journal of Aromatherapy*, 1992 vol. 4 no. 2.

Ylinen, J. and Cash, M., *Sports Massage*, Stanley Paul & Co Ltd, 1988.

GLOSSARY

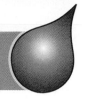

Adipose tissue – connective tissue containing fat cells.

Alimentary canal – the tube extending from the mouth to the anus.

Allergens – a substance which causes an allergy.

Allergy – an extreme sensitivity to certain substances or allergens.

Alveoli – air sacs in the lungs.

Antibody – a protein substance in the blood which is formed by lymphocytes to combat disease.

Antigens – a substance which stimulates the production of antibodies.

Appendicular skeleton – the bones of the limbs and the two girdles.

Arterioles – small branches of arteries which end in capillaries.

Autonomic nervous system – the part of the nervous system that regulates the internal organs, made up of the sympathetic and parasympathetic divisions. The effects of each counteract and balance the effects of the other.

Axilla – the armpit.

Axial skeleton – the central part of the skeleton, skull, vertebral column and bones of the trunk.

Ayurvedic – A traditional Indian healing system to balance mind, body and spirit.

B-cell – White blood cell that produces antibodies in response to an antigen.

Bonding – closeness of a child to its mother or father.

Bronchioles – small tubes in the lung leading to the alveoli.

Capillary – very small blood vessels which connect the arteries and veins.

Cartilage – tough, flexible connective tissue found in parts of the body needing firm support.

Cellulite – subcutaneous fat causing dimpling of the skin.

Cellulitis – inflammation of subcutaneous connective tissue.

Closed question – a question that can be answered with a simple yes or no.

Collagen – tough, inelastic material which is a constituent of connective tissue and bone.

Connective tissue – containing different types of cells and fibres, it holds other tissues and organs together and gives them support.

Contraindication – a condition indicating that a treatment must not be carried out.

Dermis – the deep layer of the skin containing blood vessels, nerves, glands, hair roots and connective tissue.

Desquamation – the removal of the surface cells of the skin.

Dextrous – the skilful, precise use of the hands.

Diffusion – a method of evenly spreading fine droplets of a fluid into the air.

Distal – the furthest point of a limb from the body.

Diuretic – causing increased passing of urine.

Effleurage – stroking massage movements in the direction of venous and lymphatic flow.

Endocrine glands – those glands that produce chemical messengers (hormones) which are carried in the blood stream and are responsible for maintaining homeostasis.

Enzyme – a protein substance acting as a catalyst for chemical reactions in the body.

Epidermis – the tough outer layer of the skin which protects the deeper tissues.

Erythema – a superficial redness of the skin.

Friction – a brisk rubbing of the skin to produce warmth.

Gluteal – the region over the buttocks.

Hazard – danger.

Histamine – a chemical substance released by the mast cells in the skin as a result of irritation, causing itching, redness and weals.

Holism – a concept of health which includes the whole person, physical, psychological, and emotional.

Homeostasis – the maintenance of the internal environment of the body.

Hormone – the chemical messengers produced by the endocrine glands.

Hygiene – the state of cleanliness, environmental and personal.

Keratin – insoluble protein which is the main component of hair and nails.

Ligament – band of tough inelastic connective tissue joining bone to bone at joints.

Limbic system – a part of the brain closely related to the thalamus and hypothalamus thought to affect the emotions.

Lymph – a yellowish fluid contained in the lymphatic vessels. It is similar to tissue fluid but contains more protein.

Lymph nodes – often called lymph glands, they are small bean-shaped bodies situated along lymph vessels which filter the lymph and make lymphocytes and antibodies.

Lymphocytes – white blood cells which make antibodies to destroy bacteria or viruses.

Mailshot – letters sent to a large number of customers as an advertisement.

Meridian – A pathway in the body along which energy is said to flow.

Metabolic rate – the amount of energy used by a body in a set time.

NCVQ – National Council for Vocational Qualifications.

Open questions – questions which cannot be answered with a simple yes or no.

Osteopathy – method of treatment by manipulation.

Palliative – relieving pain or helping a problem without dealing with the cause.

Patch test – application to a small patch of skin of a substance suspected of causing a reaction.

Patella – kneecap.

Peristalsis – the rhythmic muscular movement of the bowel which moves food onwards.

Petrissage – massage movements which involve pressing and squeezing the tissues.

pH value – acidity/alkalinity maintained at a constant level in the body.

Physiotherapy – the treatment of disease, disability or injury by physical means.

Phytohormones – hormone-like substances found in plants.

Popliteal – the area at the back of the knee.

Prone – lying face down.

Proximal – the part of a limb closest to the body.

Receptors – sensory structures receiving stimuli.

Reflex – an involuntary response to a stimulus.

Renal – relating to the kidneys.

Rolling – massage movements where the tissues are rolled between thumb and fingers.

Sedative – slows down activity.

Shiatsu – a method of physical treatment involving pressures on certain points of the body.

Stress – psychological pressure caused by situations or other people.

Supine – lying face up.

Synergy – working together to the benefit of each.

Synovial – relating to the synovial membrane that surrounds freely moveable joints and which produces synovial fluid.

T-cell – Lymphocyte active in immunity, matures in the thymus gland and destroys foreign cells direct.

Tapotement – massage movements that involve tapping or percussion on the body.

Tendon – tough bands of inelastic connective tissue linking muscle to bone.

Tension – the body's reaction to stress.

Therapy – any form of treatment.

Thrombus – a clot of blood in the heart or blood vessels.

Toxin – any substance which causes damage to tissues.

Traction – gentle stretching of a part, especially related to joints.

Ulnar – the little finger side of the arm or hand.

Urinary – related to the function of the bladder.

Venule – the small veins which are the termination of the venous system.

Volatile – substances that may be vaporised into the atmosphere.

Equipment (treatment couches and accessories)

Carlton Professional
Carlton House,
Commerce Way
Lancing
West Sussex BN15 8TA
Tel: 01903 761100

Marshcouch
14, Robinsfield
Hemel Hempstead
Herts HP1 1RW
Tel: 01442 263 199

New Concept
2 Bermuda Road
Ransomes Euro Park
Ipswich,
Suffolk IP3 9RU
Tel: 01473 721559

Polmac Enterprises (Storage boxes)
3, The Briars
High Wycombe,
Bucks. HP1 1ED
Tel: 01494 533857

Oils

Bay House Aromatics (also burners)
88, St Georges Rd.
Brighton BN2 1EE
Tel: 01273 601109

Essentially Oils
8-10 Mount Farm
Junction Road
Churchill
Chipping Norton OX7 6NP
Tel: 01608 659 544

Neal's Yard Remedies
15 Neal's Yard
Covent Garden
London WC2H 9DP
Tel: 020 7379 7222
or by mail order:
29 John Dalton Street
Manchester M2 62S
Tel: 0161 831 7875

Saffron Oils
Belmont House
Newport
Saffron Walden
Essex CB11 3RF
Tel: 01799 540622

Associations

The Association of Reflexologists
27 Old Gloucester Street
London WC1N 3XX
Tel: 0870 5673 320
www.aor.org.uk

Aromatherapy Organisations Council
PO Box 19834
London SE25 6WF
020 8251 7912
www.aromatherapy-uk.org

British Association of Beauty Therapy and Cosmetology
BABTAC House
70 Eastgate St.
Gloucester GL1 1QN
Tel:01452 421114
www.babtac.com

British Complementary Medicine Association (BCMA)
Kensington House
33 Imperial Square
Cheltenham GL50 1QZ
01242 519911
www.BCMA.co.uk

Shiatsu Society of the UK
Eastlands Court
St Peter's Road
Rugby
Warwickshire CV21 3QP
Tel: 0178 855 5051
www.shiatsu.org

Journals

Complementary Therapies in Nursing and Midwifery
Harcourt Publishers Ltd
Foots Cray High St.
Sidcup
Kent DA14 5HP
Tel: 020 8308 5700

Health and Beauty Salon
Quadrant House
The Quadrant
Sutton
Surrey SM2 5AS
020 8652 8268

The International Journal of Aromatherapy
Harcourt Publishers Ltd
Foots Cray High Street
Sidcup
Kent DA14 5HP
Tel: 020 8308 5700

INDEX

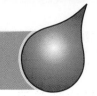

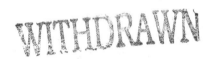